TECHNIQUES
OF
INNER
HEALING

Also by D. Scott Rogo

An Experience of Phantoms
Beyond Reality: The Role Unseen Dimensions Play in Our Lives
Exploring Psychic Phenomena: Beyond Mind and Matter
Leaving the Body: A Practical Guide to Astral Projection
Life After Death: The Case for Survival of Bodily Death
Miracles: A Scientific Exploration of Wondrous Phenomena
NAD: A Study of Some Unusual Other World Experiences, Vol. I
NAD: Psychic Study of the Music of the Spheres, Vol. II
On the Track of the Poltergeist
Our Psychic Potentials
Parapsychology: A Century of Inquiry
Psychic Breakthroughs Today
*The Infinite Boundary: Spirit Possession, Madness, and Multiple
    Personality*
The Poltergeist Experience
*The Search for Yesterday: A Critical Examination of the Evidence for
    Reincarnation*
The Welcoming Silence

NEW TECHNIQUES OF

INNER HEALING

D. SCOTT ROGO

PARAGON HOUSE
NEW YORK

First edition, 1992

Published in the United States by

Paragon House
90 Fifth Avenue
New York, N.Y. 10011

The eleven interviews that appear in this book were originally published in *Science of Mind* magazine between 1986 and 1989.

Library of Congress Cataloging-in-Publishing Data

Rogo, D. Scott.
    New techniques of inner healing / D. Scott Rogo. — 1st ed.
        p.   cm.
    Includes bibliographical references.
    ISBN 1-55778-444-2 — ISBN 1-55778-492-2 (pbk.)
    1. Alternative medicine. I. Title.
R733.R63   1992
615.5'3 — dc20   91-20983
                                                            CIP

Manufactured in the United States of America
10 9 8 7 6 5 4 3 2 1

TABLE OF CONTENTS

FOREWORD

Healing and growth would certainly top the list of catchwords linked to New Age thinking. These two concepts have literally guided this cultural phenomenon since its inception and gradual rise. New Age thinking and living show people that in order for us to grow, we must first overcome our psychological, emotional, and perhaps physical wounds. These are the psychic scars we sustained through faulty upbringing and materialistic cultural values, and that we continue to suffer through the emotional setbacks everyone confronts during day-to-day living.

Growth and recovery from inner pain represent the central topics discussed in these pages. Between 1986 and 1989 I was engaged in a novel project in collaboration with *Science of Mind* magazine, the official organ of the United Church of Religious Science. Overcoming our past and current conditioning and inner pain can be difficult without proper guidance. Seeing the need for this form of input, I began interviewing renowned experts on human growth and inner healing for the magazine. These high-profile individuals have specialized in dealing with such problems as stress in the workplace, grief and bereavement, painful childhood experiences, and so forth. The tools they espouse range from boosting the immune system through positive emotional experience, to coping strategies in the face of personal crisis, to the healing power of music.

But these conversations extend beyond the typical "power" of positive thinking banalities. The people I interviewed were specifically chosen because they recognize the limitations that beset conventional psychology. We cannot help people psychologically *unless* we speak to their spiritual concerns. So each of the interviews in this book combines hints for psychological healing with suggestions for spiritual discovery and growth. Some of them suggest that this process of inner growth can be a healing pathway by itself.

Unlike many of the interviews published in popular magazines, these interviews were extremely structured. While first contemplating this project, I was forced to confront the following issue: Why do most interviews seem so tedious? I concluded that the reason was fairly simple. Few interviewers really study what their journalistic subjects and guests have said, thought, and written. So before each interview was undertaken, I read the books, scientific papers, and several previous interviews on each expert. This general "process of familiarization" gave me the tools to structure each discussion on selected issues carefully chosen to best interest the reading public. The result has been a collection of discussions and interviews with little fluff or irrelevancies.

The goal of each conversation was geared toward the practical side of the contributor's work or research. In other words, a portion of every interview covers the way by which the contributor's insights can be put to practical use by the reader. These conversations were not designed as exercises in intellectual self-indulgence, but to give the reader tools and methods to improve his or her everyday life. What resulted were interviews ranging over several unrelated subjects but which seemed to focus on a central theme: that overcoming the scars of the past and present promises us spiritual and psychological growth for the future.

D. Scott Rogo
August 1990

INTRODUCTION—
SPIRITUALITY, HEALTH,
AND THE MIND

Probably everybody reading these pages knows the power of the "placebo" effect. Sometimes totally inert substances, such as pills filled with sugar, have remarkable effects upon the body... but only if the patient believes in their efficacy. The basis of the effect is the simple power of suggestion: that deep within us lies the power of the brain to trick the body into responding to its (the mind's) commands. Psychological suggestion has long been one of psychology's most powerful tools and constitutes the mysterious phenomenon by which hypnosis and some forms of religious healing (not to mention psychotherapy) work. But the power of suggestion can influence the body in ways even some psychologists would find remarkable.

I learned this lesson one fall day in Los Angeles, when the environmental pollen counts were driving everyone in the city crazy. I'm lucky that I don't suffer from hypersensitivity responses (commonly known as allergies) to the pollens which pervade our beautiful—but sometimes smoggy—California skies. But the pollen counts that fall had been especially dense and everyone in the San Fernando Valley (a suburb of Los Angeles) was succumbing to sneezing, scratchy throats, and watering eyes. I was so miserable that I finally called my family physician to get some medication which (unlike over-the-counter antihistamines) wouldn't make me sleepy. I took the first pill while riding the bus to pick up my car, which was in the shop for some minor repairs. Every symptom I was suffering lifted within minutes.

I was extremely impressed by the medication and, weeks later,

2   explained to my doctor how well the pills worked. He was skeptical of my story and replied that the drug I took invariably takes three days to build up in the blood to a therapeutic dose. It couldn't have worked that fast, he emphasized.

What had really occurred was relatively simple. Somehow I mentally influenced my immune system so that certain cells in my body—i.e., mast cells in the tissues and basophils in the blood—stopped releasing histamine and other chemicals upon binding with the pollen. It was a pure case of *psychoneuroimmunology*, the power of the brain to regulate the body's immune defenses, a discipline coming to the forefront of medicine's new frontiers. It was certainly a minor case of this surprising phenomenon, for more impressive cases of this same effect can certainly be found in the literature of both psychology and medicine. For example, some experts believe that our power to fight even cancer is inherently related to psychological factors. Now the model for cancer proposed by psychoneuroimmunologists is not universally accepted by oncologists, but more and more experts seem to be taking it seriously.

Cancer cells do not represent powerful invaders within the body—pouncing upon the body's organs, setting up swarming growths, and multiplying without regulation. Cancer cells are biologically confused cells, being nothing more than mutations from the body's previously healthy blood or tissues. The reasons for these mutations remain basically unknown. (Viral invasion of healthy cells seems to play a role in some cancers, while other mechanisms, including chance, probably lie at the root of others.) The concept of "immune surveillance" states that the body is probably constantly producing cancer cells, eliminated as a matter of course by certain blood cells genetically programmed to seek them out and destroy them. It has been suggested that curious cells called Natural Killer Cells serve this purpose. Of course, other mechanisms within the incredible complex machinery of the immune system undoubtedly play a contributing role in this regulation.*

If the theory of immune surveillance is correct, it makes sense that

---

*For a detailed explanation of the mechanics by which psychological processes influence both the endocrine system and the immune system, a fine start would be Dr. Ernest L. Rossi's *The Psychobiology of Mind-Body Healing: New Concepts of Therapeutic Hypnosis.* (New York: Norton, 1986)

mental processes can influence cancer... either keeping us safe or by
leading us to fall prey to the disease. Now this isn't saying that psychological factors either cause or can cure cancer. It merely means
that psychological and situational factors probably interplay with
genetic predisposition, environmental pollution, and other factors
which contribute to cancer.

In this respect, there exists a large body of evidence that some
cancers relate to psychological crisis. For example, take a look at the
following studies on the effects of severe life changes on the onset of
cancer:

- As far back as the 1930s, French cancer specialists realized
  that the disease could be catalyzed by emotional trauma.
- The eminent psychologist Dr. Bruno Klupfer found that cancer
  developed more rapidly in patients struggling with emotional
  upsets.
- Back in the 1960s, Dr. Lawrence LeShan in New York discovered that widowed or divorced people had a greater chance of
  developing cancer than married or single persons. This finding
  led Dr. LeShan to suggest that people suffering from severe loss
  are likely to develop the disease in response.
- In a follow-up study, LeShan and Dr. E. R. Worthington discovered that sixty-two percent of their cancer patients developed
  their illnesses shortly after losing a spouse or other significant
  person in their lives.

So much for merely a *few* of the studies on situational crisis and its
influence on cancer. Now let's briefly go a step further and examine
personality factors that influence the disease.

Why is it that some people develop cancer and immediately suc-
cumb to its ravages, while other people—even with spreading cancer—learn to control and survive the condition? Instead of looking at
people particularly prone to the disease, let's be more optimistic.
Let's look at people with the uncanny knack of *beating* the condition.

The personality of the "exceptional cancer patient" (the previously
called long-term survivor) was first described by a team of
researchers headed by Dr. Jeanne Achterberg, a brilliant psychologist then working in Texas. Their research was published in 1977 in
the journal *Psychotherapy: Theory, Research and Practice.* Dr.

4   Achterberg and her colleagues followed a group of cancer patients diagnosed as having less than a year to live, and critically examined those patients who survived a year longer. By comparing their scores on several conventional psychology tests to those of the patients who died on schedule, the Texas researchers isolated several factors that contributed to the survival of the former group. The psychologists typified these patients as "more creative, more receptive to new ideas, flexible and argumentative. Often they were down-right ornery." Notable, too, was the fact that these survivors placed more stock in relying upon inner resources than outside support while battling their illness. They also resisted their initial, terminal diagnoses and took a combative stance toward their life-threatening diseases.

The subjects in this study did not represent a random sample, though. They tended to be college-educated, white, and financially secure. Would cancer patients from less successful or more economically disadvantaged communities conform to these personality patterns? This issue has been explored by some research undertaken by researchers with the Parkland Memorial Hospital of the South Western Medical School in Dallas. The cancer patients in this study tended to be poor, racially mixed, and several were drawing upon public assistance. After completing the study, the profile of the long-term cancer survivor in this study turned out to be different from the exceptional patients of Dr. Achterberg. The people who "beat the odds" in this study tended to look outside of themselves for support when their medical crises struck. They looked to their jobs, to their churches, and to personal relationships to help them fight cancer. For women suffering from metastasized breast cancer, for example, a good relationship with their husbands was necessary for their long-term survival.

Dr. Achterberg, who currently teaches at the Institute for Transpersonal Psychology in San Francisco, thinks she understands why the findings of these studies were partially contradictory. Writing in her excellent book *Imagery in Healing: Shamanism and Modern Medicine,* she points out that: "A San Francisco psychiatrist who has worked with cancer patients for a long time believes that the patients who do well already knew how to fight before they were diagnosed. I think it is absolutely correct, although no one has ever studied the issue systematically. People who have been in difficult straits and escaped from them have learned to rally their defenses and tested their resources. They have already identified a resource system." In other words, people from different socioeconomic strata naturally learn different coping strategies for stressful events in their lives.

The moral of the story is that there is no single way to fight a life-threatening disease. Whether a person turns inward to mobilize his or her inner resources or turns to their family and Church will be based on their past life experiences. But these studies seem to show that by relying on a support system—any system—perhaps a person can "beat the odds" when facing a serious illness.

So far, nothing I've been saying should strike the reader as surprising. The past few pages have merely recapitulated what any book on psychoneuroimmunology would posit.

But now let's take the science of psychoneuroimmunology a step further. Could there be an X factor in the body which plays a role in even more radical recovery from disease... some "force" that neither science nor psychology has officially recognized?

One of the most impressive cases of a "cure through suggestion" ever recorded was originally published in 1957 by Dr. Bruno Klupfer, whose research on the psychology of cancer was briefly mentioned earlier in this chapter. Dr. Klupfer was an expert in the study and use of the famous Rorschach Ink Blot test. (This is the famous examination by which a person's psychological profile can be evaluated by way of his or her responses to a series of blotches.) Dr. Klupfer reported the case in his presidential speech to the Society for Projective Techniques and it has since become a classic in the literature. The remarkable story centers on a patient merely named Mr. Wright and was reported to the researcher by the former's physician, Dr. Philip West.

The patient was originally diagnosed with lymphosarcoma, a cancer in the lymph system which severely impairs the body's immune system and can become life-threatening. Serious tumors had formed throughout the patient's body and by the time the patient was treated by Dr. West, he was suffering from anemia, which is a common side effect of this form of cancer. The disease was so advanced that nobody in the clinic where he lay bedridden thought he could survive even if treated for the cancer. Dr. West, however, was more optimistic, for he had recently read of a new "wonder" drug for cancer called Krebiozen and clinical trials of the medication were scheduled to begin in his own clinic. Even though the patient was too close to

6   death to take part in the trials, he begged for the drug and Dr. West—after some consideration—gave him an injection one Friday. By the following Monday, Mr. Wright's cancer had gone into complete remission!

"I had left him feeble, gasping for air, completely bedridden," explains the physician. "Now here he was walking around the ward, chatting happily with the nurses, and spreading his message of good cheer to any who would listen."

Mr. Wright's tumors had nearly disappeared "like snowballs on a hot stove." The change was much more remarkable than his radiation treatments could have produced.

Dr. West was suspicious of the improvement, though. Other patients in the hospital were receiving injections of the same medication and showing little response to it. Despite his skepticism, the physician continued giving the patient Krebiozen injections and watching his improvement, much to his bewilderment. The patient was seemingly cured of his cancer in ten days.

The upshot to the story came two months later when news reports were circulated that the clinical trials on Krebiozen had failed and that the drug simply didn't work. Mr. Wright's optimism and faith in the drug faltered when he read the news, and his lymphoma returned. The patient was rehospitalized in as serious a condition as ever.

Dr. West realized by this time that some aspect of his patient's mind was controlling his disease, so he decided to try an experiment. He falsely told Mr. Wright that Krebiozen had lost its effectiveness only because its "shelf life" was extremely limited and the original batch had deteriorated. Then he offered to give Mr. Wright an injection of a new and improved version of Krebiozen that was double the strength of the original. The patient became ecstatic over the news and eagerly took the injection... of simple water!

"Recovery from his second near-terminal state was even more dramatic than the first," reported the physician. "Tumor masses melted, chest fluid vanished, and he became ambulatory, and even went back to flying again."

The denouement to the case occurred sometime later, when the American Medical Association publicly disclosed that Krebiozen was worthless as a cancer drug. Mr. Wright heard the news, became depressed, and died within a week from the cancer that originally hospitalized him.

But what was special about Mr. Wright that he should respond so spectacularly to the drug, even while other people in the same clinic failed to react? We will never know the complete reason, but some hints were offered by Bruno Klupfer on the basis of the patient's Rorschach responses.

Klupfer found that the patient lacked a strong sense of self. This left Mr. Wright with considerable energy to invest in his faith in the Krebiozen. This investment was a superficial one, however, and was destroyed by the news of the medication's inefficacy. Dr. Klupfer explained to the Society for Projective Techniques that the patient's psychological investment in the drug "could not last since it was not reinforced by any deep-rooted personality center with a long-range point of view which could have counteracted the catastrophic effect of his disappointment about the drug." The psychologist emphasized his point by way of a metaphor. "While he was floating along on the surface of the water—the influence of his optimistic auto-suggestion or suggestion," explained Dr. Klupfer, "he was transformed into a heavy stone and sank to the bottom without resistance at the moment when the power of suggestion expired."

Now I am personally far from sure that Dr. Klupfer has given us the final solution to the strange case of Mr. Wright. Why didn't the patient respond similarly to the other treatments he received in the earlier course of his disease? I think most cancer specialists and immunologists would concur that the phenomenal rate of Mr. Wright's recovery is more than the recuperative powers of the body can explain. Somehow these powers were radically enhanced by some power upon which the patient drew.

The famous case of Mr. Wright has been reported several times in books on the mind/body relationship, but I feel that most experts miss the point of the story. The case is generally used to illustrate the phenomenal power of the placebo. I believe that the real message is that, deep within the mind, *each of us possesses some unknown power upon which we can draw to cure even life-threatening illnesses.*

Remember that Mr. Wright wasn't merely sick when he took the Krebiozen, he was literally at the portal of death. But his "faith" saved him until it was countermanded by his own bitter disillusionment in the drug. It is up to psychology, medicine, and religion to explore the dynamics of this faith or power, so that we can learn to harness and employ it in our everyday lives.

8   This issue is, in fact, one of the central themes of this book: Is there some healing power linked to the mind and body upon which we can draw? This possibility gives rise to several secondary issues:

- Can this power or potential be used to heal us psychologically as well as physically?
- Are there specific techniques we can use to establish contact with this power?
- Can this power be beneficially projected to others?
- Can we establish wholeness within ourselves by touching, praying, or otherwise healing people dear to us?

I am certainly not the first person to raise these issues, which emerge from the psychological study of the placebo effect. Probably the most famous book ever written on the placebo and the role it plays in psychological change and healing is Jerome Frank's classic *Persuasion and Healing: A Comparative Study of Psychotherapy.* Dr. Frank is a psychiatrist at the Johns Hopkins School of Medicine in Baltimore. On page seventy-four of his book he illustrated the incredible power of the placebo by showing its role in faith healing:

> The apparent success of healing methods based on various ideologies and methods compels the conclusion that the healing power of faith resides in the patient's state of mind, not in the validity of its object. At the risk of laboring this point, an experimental demonstration of it with three severely ill, bedridden women may be reported. One had chronic inflammation of the gall bladder with stones, the second had failed to recuperate from a major abdominal operation and was practically a skeleton, and the third was dying of widespread cancer. The physician first permitted a prominent local faith healer to try to cure them by absent treatment without the patients' knowledge. Nothing happened. Then he told the patients about the faith healer, built up their expectations over several days, and finally assured them that he would be treating them from a distance at a certain time the next day. This was a time in which he was sure that the healer did *not* work. At the suggested time all three patients improved quickly and dramatically. The second was permanently cured. The other two were not, but showed striking temporary responses. The cancer patient, who was severely anemic and whose tissues had become waterlogged, promptly excreted all the accumulated fluid, recovered from her anemia, and regained sufficient strength to go home and resume her household duties. She remained virtually symptom-free until her death.

The gall balder patient lost her symptoms, went home, and had no recurrence for several years. These three patients were greatly helped by a belief that was false—that the faith healer was treating them from a distance—suggesting that "expectant trust" in itself can be a powerful healing force.

But the eminent Dr. Frank is honest enough not to stop with such cases. For on the very next page of his book, the psychiatrist warns his readers not to take a purely reductionistic stance toward faith healing on the basis of the placebo effect.

"One cannot conclude this review of nonmedical healing without mentioning the possibility that some individuals... may have a gift of healing that defies scientific explanation," Dr. Frank points out. "Nor can one rule out the possibility—indeed the evidence for it is quite persuasive—that some healers serve as a kind of conduit for a healing force in the universe, often called the life force, that, for want of a better term, must be called supernatural."

Whether this force lies within the universe or within the mind is a fascinating point of debate. But it is to the nature of this healing power that I would like to turn next.

MESMERISM AND THE LIFE FORCE

When and where the concept of a universal "life force" first evolved in the West is a matter of conjecture. This sort of thinking was first *popularized*, at least, by Sir Kenelm Digby (1603–1665) in England. A sometime writer, diplomat, and naval commander, Digby continually oscillated in his religious beliefs and was expelled from England in 1643 upon his release from prison for his political sympathies. He returned to the islands when the Royalists were overthrown and worked there for Catholic interests. But by that time, his fascination had turned to the occult. Whether he was a mountebank or genuinely interested in the healing arts isn't known, but he later developed a "powder of sympathy," which (purportedly) contained the power to heal over great distances. When a friend was injured in a duel, for instance, it is said that Digby was given the blood-stained garter which had bound the sufferer's hand. Digby placed the powder in some water and then soaked the garter... whereupon the wounded friend—whose back was turned during the operation—suddenly pronounced himself healed! He explained that "a pleasant kind of fresh-

10   ness" spread over his hand when the garter was immersed in the water.

Later that night (presumably at his home), Digby removed the garter and let it dry. Soon a servant came running in, shouting that the patient's hands were burning like they were "between coals of fire." Digby reimmersed the garter, which provided great relief to the patient.

The truth or fiction of this story is impossible to decipher, but it illustrates the popular notion that some sort of life force exists in the universe. This ever pervading force can be tapped by people or funneled into physical substances. It was upon this latter tradition that Digby worked when he claimed he possessed a salve that could cure a wound, even without ever touching it.

But even Sir Kenelm's claims were not novel. The precursors to this kind of thinking date back much further to the writings of such philosopher-healers as Philippus Aureolus (Theophrastus Bombastus von Hohenheim), the Swiss inconoclast who called himself Paracelsus (1493–1541). He is chiefly remembered today for his observation that the physician's job is merely to set the stage for Nature to heal. Paracelsus, and many who followed in his wake, believed that healing was due in part to magnetism, then only a partially understood phenomenon of Nature. Running magnets over a patient's body to help regulate some sort of life force—which pervades the cosmos and extends into the body—became part and parcel of medical practices of the day. The philosophical rationale for such procedures was supplied by writers such as Robert Fludd (1574–1637), a British medical student who pursued his education on the Continent. When he returned to England in 1605 he set up practice as a physician. He was apparently a charismatic person and openly supported the use of magnets in his practice. Like so many intellectuals of his day, Fludd was preoccupied with theology, metaphysical philosophy, and their interface with medicine. He believed, for example, that specific demons were responsible for certain diseases. Later in life, however, he grew more enamored with cosmological models for disease and summed up his philosophy in his *Philosophia Moysaica* published in 1637.

Fludd's theory was that the human body, the stars, and every physical substance radiate beams of force interacting with each other. The influence of the stars is, however, preeminent and it is the interplay of these beams that regulates life and its blights. Medicine was merely the skill of manipulating such forces through chemistry and, sometimes, with lodestones to balance these forces in the body.

This general conceptual model was called the *magnetic philosophy*. While perhaps it sounds like superstitious drivel, this type of thinking has persisted in different guises right up to the present day. Even such practices as *therapeutic touch* (see the interview with Dr. Janet Quinn later in the book) build on a related premise.

The magnetic school of philosophy had several notable enthusiasts, including John Baptist van Helmont, who was born into a noble Brabantian family in 1557. A true renaissance man of his time, van Helmont was first drawn to mathematics and physics before becoming a physician in 1599. Most of his time was devoted to experimental chemistry, but he is best remembered for deciphering the physiology of the stomach. Soon, though, he became engrossed in studying the existence of life forces in the universe, and whether physicians could harnass them. He eventually came to the conclusion that the body is itself a magnet and that sickness could be overcome by manipulating and channeling such forces in and through the patient. Lodestones and the power of the physician's will were the physician's key tools and van Helmont canvassed the countryside practicing his healing skills, often offering his services to the local townfolk free of charge.

The proverbial stage was now set for the rise of the Mesmeric movement, which popularized such teachings by bringing them to the public's attention. Mesmerism was named for its discoverer, Franz Anton Mesmer (1734–1815), who was born in a small community near the German shore of Lake Constance. Little is known about his childhood, but later in life, he entered the Jesuit Theological School in Dillingen. He was an intellectually restless youth, and by 1759 he was studying law in Vienna, but then switched to medicine. He completed his degree in 1766 with a dissertation concerning the influence of the planets on human sickness. By the time he earned his medical degree, he was thirty-three years old.

Becoming established as a physician in Vienna wasn't difficult for Mesmer. His marriage in 1767 to a wealthy widow from the European nobility secured his entry into cultured society. There he revealed himself to be a connoisseur of the arts, and his mansion was often frequented by Leopold and the young Wolfgang Amadeus Mozart. The

12   pivotal case in Mesmer's early career was that of Franzl Oesterlin, a twenty-five-year-old hysteric who suffered from chronic pains, episodes of delirium, rage, and compulsive fainting. Today she would have been diagnosed as mentally ill, but such insights were not to come to Vienna for over a century with the Freudian revolution. Mesmer noted in his treatment of Fraülein Oesterlin that her symptoms were periodic, which he felt was due to some sort of fluidic "tide" in her body. So he gave her a special preparation to drink and then connected magnets to specific parts of her body. The patient, resting in Mesmer's parlor, soon described wonderful streams of fluid rushing down her body and was soon "cured."

Fraülein Oesterlin was feeling so energetic, in fact, that she soon married Mesmer's stepson! Based on his success with Fraülein Oesterlin, Mesmer developed his theory of an ever present life force in the universe that could both cause and cure disease. The Viennese physician couldn't believe that his cure was solely due to magnets, and postulated that they were only secondary to this more basic force, which he dubbed *animal magnetism.* This subtle fluid, Mesmer posited, pervades the entire universe but specifically accumulates in the body. Mesmer would spend the rest of his life studying this strange life force.

The prompt and sensational cure of Fraülein Oesterlin secured Mesmer's reputation and he was subsequently invited by the Baron Horeczky de Horka to visit his castle in Slovakia. The poor baron was suffering from a convulsive disorder and hoped Mesmer could cure him.

By this time, Mesmer had come to the conclusion that magnets were superfluous. Whatever the nature of the life force, he believed he could control it simply with rods or his hands—by moving them in certain directions over the body. This force could be expelled, if necessary, by shaking the hands upon completion of the "pass." Such procedures were looked upon with suspicion by the medical establishment, to say the least, and even Baron de Horka resisted Mesmer for several days.

But the physician was an imposing figure in his gold-embroidered gray robe. With one foot placed in a water-filled bucket to ground himself, Mesmer stood by the patient while a servant ran an iron rod—supported from the bottom of the same bucket—up and down the patient. The appreciative baron reported feeling much better with his "fluid" correctly regulated, but the cure was undermined when the nobleman's own doctor showed up and suggested that it would probably be only temporary. The baron fell victim to his physician's suggestions and refused further treatment.

In his curious and honest response to the situation, Mesmer refused payment from the baron, explaining that he (the baron) was not cured and needed further sessions. If nothing else, this conclusion to the de Horka imbroglio reveals that Mesmer was more than the cheap charlatan, as history tends to portray him.

Despite his failure with the baron, Mesmer's visit to Slovakia lasted thirteen weeks, during which he treated dozens of sick in the manor. Through the use of his mesmeric passes, he cured a deaf man, a convulsive, and even demonstrated that the life force could work over distance. This phenomenon serves as a fascinating story in itself:

The incident began when some of the baron's friends and a Herr Seyfert—tutor to the nobleman's children—experimented to see if Mesmer could influence a person in a separate room. In order to test this extravagant notion, they took a patient suffering from spasms into a second room, separated from them by a brick wall. Mesmer merely pointed his finger in the direction of the patient. When he moved his finger horizontally, the patient's spasms increased. When the physician made circular movements in the air, they completely ceased. Mesmer wasn't surprised by the results, explaining to Seyfert and the others that the magnetic fluid could easily pass through physical matter.

When news of these demonstrations spread, Mesmer's reputation in Europe was insured, much to the chagrin of the Viennese medical establishment, who naturally feared that Mesmer would undercut their practices. Mesmer, in the meantime, returned to the shores of Lake Constance in July 1775 and continued to reap success after success with his cures. He was even nominated that year to the Bavarian Academy of Science, but a public scandal was soon to follow.

This curious chapter in Mesmer's life began when he took the sightless eighteen-year-old Theresia Paradis into his Vienna home for treatment. The girl was somewhat of a celebrity despite her handicap. With the help of embossed teaching materials secured by her wealthy family, she had received a formidable and refined education. She

14   later became a prodigy with her needlework and with her piano
recitals. Mesmer worked with the girl at her family's request and her
sight began to return; but Paradis's physician was outraged and
denied the improvement... successfully provoking Theresia's family
into a feud with Mesmer. Her treatments with Mesmer were discontinued and Theresia's sight was permanently lost. The Viennese medical fraternity exploited the scandal and charged Mesmer with charla-
tanry, while he and his followers replied that the failure was due to
the interference of the Paradis family. Since young Theresia was
earning her living as a blind prodigy with the generous patronage of
the Empress Maria Theresa, the family had a vested interest in keeping her blind. Regaining her sight would have been socially and
financially disastrous for them.

Whatever the truth of the matter, Mesmer decided to leave Vienna.
There is some evidence that he suffered from a serious depression,
from which he only gradually emerged, charismatic as ever. Infused
now with a rekindled desire to make his discoveries known, he set
out for Paris in the early part of 1778.

Paris was a more restless city than complacent Vienna, most likely
due to the instability of the French monarchy and the hedonistic life-
style of the upper classes. Parisian society tended to take up every
fad that came its way and was the perfect social setting for Mesmer to
spread his secular gospel. Settling himself in a private residence, the
physician from Lake Constance soon enjoyed a thriving practice, but
he also introduced some important changes into his work. From the
treatment of individual clients, Mesmer graduated to group magnetic
sessions with the introduction of his new innovation: the *baquet*. This
was a device specifically invented to channel the life force. It consisted of a large tub piled with bottles of magnetized liquid and then
filled with additional water. A lid was placed over the barrel with
openings from which metal rods protruded. The clients sat around the
baquet and were connected by a rope. These clients came to be treated for a number of conditions including, more often than not, nervous
disorders. They held the rods to their bodies in order to infuse themselves with the baquet's power, or Mesmer's minions would undertake
the job. Mesmer would usually make a regal entrance during the session wearing flowing robes and holding a wand. While the clients
magnetized themselves from the baquet, he would exhort and point
his rod at them. The results were little less than mass hysteria, from

which many people emerged—not surprisingly—cured of their problems.

An excellent description of these sessions has been left to posterity by J. P. F. Deleuze, the librarian of the Jardin des Plantes, who chronicled the Mesmeric movement in 1843:

> No diseases offensive to the sight were treated, such as sores, wens or deformities. The patients then drew near each other, touching hands, arms, knees or feet. The handsomest, youngest and most robust magnetizers held also an iron rod with which they touched the dilatory or stubborn patients. The rods and ropes had all undergone a preparation, and in a very short space of time the patients felt the magnetic influence.
>
> The women, being the most easily affected, were almost at once seized with fits of yawning and stretching; their eyes were closed, their legs gave way, and they seemed to suffocate. In vain did musical glasses and harmonicas resound, the piano and voices re-echo, these supposed aids only seemed to increase the patients' convulsive movements. Sardonic laughter, piteous moans and torrents of tears burst forth on all sides. The bodies were thrown back in spasmodic jerks, the respirations sounded like death rattles, the most terrifying symptoms were exhibited. Then suddenly the actors of this strange scene would frantically or rapturously rush towards each other, either rejoicing and embracing or thrusting away their neighbors with every appearance of horror.

Later in the session, the charismatic Dr. Mesmer would undertake to personally magnetize clients. To once more cite Delueze's fascinating descriptions:

> Mesmer, wearing a coat of lilac silk, walked up and down amid the palpitating crowd, together with D'eslon and his associates, whom he chose for their youth and comeliness. Mesmer carried a long iron wand, with which he touched the bodies of the patients, and especially those parts which were diseased; often, laying aside the wand, he magnetized them with his eyes, fixing his gaze on theirs, or applying his hands to the hypochondriac region and to the lower part of the abdomen. This application was often continued for hours, and at other times the master made use of passes. He began by placing himself *en rapport* with his subject. Seated opposite to him, foot against foot, knee against knee, he laid his fingers on the hypochrondriac region, and moved them to and fro, lightly touching the ribs. Magnetization with strong currents was substituted for these manipulations when more energetic results were to be produced. The master, erecting his fingers in a pyramid, passed his hands all over the

16   patient's body, beginning with the head, and going down over the shoulders to the feet. He then returned again, to the head, both back and front, to the belly and the back; he renewed the process again and again, until the magnetized person was saturated with the healing fluid, and was transported with pain or pleasure, both sensations being equally salutory.

While these descriptions make Mesmer seem like a huckster, there is little doubt that he sincerely believed in his magnetic force. He even tried to form liaisons with France's scientific establishment to further explore its nature.

By the late 1770s, in fact, Mesmer had operationalized his concept of the magnetic force into four basic principles:

1. It is a subtle fluid that permeates the universe and links mankind to the cosmos and to each other.
2. Disease results from an imbalance of this energy within the body. *
3. Through specific operations, the fluid can be channeled or stored so that it can be infused into people.
4. The infusion of the force into the body leads to a crisis by which the patient is cured.

Of course, the skeptic would merely argue that Mesmer primarily treated psychosomatic or psychiatric disorders. The crisis, in this regard, was just a catharsis in which the patient was cured by suggestion.

Even in Mesmer's day, skeptics were eager to discredit the concept of a universal life force as a factor in disease. They were especially vocal in France's conservative medical establishment. (This statement is redundant, of course, since medical establishments are *invariably* conservative.) So in March of 1784, the King of France bowed to considerable pressure and ordered a commission drawn from the Académie des Sciences and the Académie de Médecine to look into Mesmer's claims. A secondary committee was sent to investigate these mesmeric claims by the Société Royale de Medecine. The committee members were drawn from Paris's scientific elite,

---

* Note the similarity to such Oriental practice as acupuncture and the concept of Ch'i energy in the body, which can cause sickness if improperly balanced. The fact that such similar notions have cropped up in separate cultures is interesting, to say the least, and perhaps points to some unrecognized factor in biology and medicine.

including: the astronomer and statesman Dr. Jean Bailly, the inventive and sadly infamous Dr. Guillotine, and Benjamin Franklin. The commission did not, however, directly work and experiment with Mesmer, who was then visiting a health spa in Belgium. The commission worked instead with Dr. Charles D'Eslon, a private physician in Paris greatly influenced by Mesmer who had set up his own practice.

It should be noted that, by this time, mesmerism had become a *movement* in Paris. Working in collaboration with a lawyer and a financial backer, Mesmer opened a school of sorts—the Société de l'Harmonie—to indoctrinate students into the secrets of the magnetic force (for a high fee, of course). This large-scale commercialization of mesmerism further threatened the status quo of the medical establishment, so a commission to look into Mesmer's claims was inevitable. So, too, were its results.

The commission met with Charles D'Eslon and watched while he worked with his patients, but they were not primarily interested in whether these people were cured. The commission was more interested in whether Mesmer had discovered a new force in nature previously untapped by science. So after learning proper mesmeric procedures by watching D'Eslon, the commission conducted their own experiments both with patients and the baquet.

The commission began by determining whether or not the baquet generated an electrical force or any other detectable energy. These experiments were failures. Next they interviewed patients who had felt emanations from the baquet's rods, but concluded that air currents in the room explained these sensations. The commission finally undertook to examine the cures reported by former patients of Mesmer and D'Eslon. The scientists ultimately rejected the importance of these cures, however, pointing out that people often recover from diseases when given opposing treatments. The fact that a person was cured upon sitting at the baquet did not mean that he or she was cured *by* the baquet, they reasoned. Reported remissions from illness could be coincidental, or the diseases the patients suffered could have been imaginary.

Probably the commission's most important findings concerned the reactions people exhibited when magnetized. Members of the commission blindfolded volunteers before pointing magnetic rods at them, but the people never reacted or entered crisis when they didn't *know* they were being treated. Other blindfolded subjects experi-

18   enced the classic "crisis" when they were told they were being magnetized, but weren't!

So after considerable effort, the commission reported back to the
King of France that magnetism was nonsense and that Mesmer
should be discredited.

Despite the report's strong conclusions, one of the committee members refused to endorse it. M. de Jessieu of the Société Royale de
Medecine had been impressed by Mesmer's and D'Eslon's patients.
In a separate statement, he pointed out to the king that some patients
reported cures of serious medical conditions that usually failed to
respond to conventional medical intervention. Dr. Jessieu noted, too,
a phenomenon that his fellow observers had overlooked. Sometimes
small muscular spasms resulted when the magnetic rods were directed toward the patients. These curious tics were displayed by subjects
unaware of the exact position of the rods. The French scientist was
impressed by these small effects and felt that they were inconsistent
with the general findings of the commission.

Despite the negative report of the commission, Mesmer and his
Société de l'Harmonie flourished and prospered. The popular press
soon entered the fray and published several reports that Mesmer's
doctrines were plagiarized from earlier philosophers and scientists.
The real challenge to Mesmer's credibility came, however, when his
own disciples rebelled and fragmented, suggesting that their mentor's
scientific models and discoveries had explanations other than a universal life force in nature.

Probably the most important of these revisionists was the kindly
Amand-Marie-Jacques de Chastenet, the Marquis de Puységur
(1751–1825) who, with his brothers, became an enthusiastic early
follower of Mesmer and his Society. A fabulously wealthy landowner,
the Marquis was scientifically inclined and compassionately concerned for the peasants who lived on his estate. While practicing
mesmerism on the local peasantry, he discovered that the magnetic
passes popularized by Mesmer sometimes placed subjects into a somnambulistic state. The dramatic crisis of the Parisian parlor room was
not the inevitable result of the procedure. This somnambulistic state
was both mysterious and wondrous, for those entering into it sometimes became clairvoyant. Everyday people could suddenly predict
the future and diagnose the illnesses of subjects brought before them.

Aside from his discovery of the somnambulistic state (renamed hypnosis by later investigators), de Puységur revised Mesmer's doctrines. He concluded that his mentor's talk of a life force or fluid in nature was perhaps only partly true or even nonsense. The true nature of the force was linked, the marquis believed, to the operator's will. Soon the insightful nobleman founded his own society, the Société Harmonique des Amis Réunis, which rejected the fluidic theory of the earlier mesmerists. This revisionist movement would probably have usurped Mesmer's influence but for the French Revolution in 1789, which diverted the French public from such metaphysical debates. Although he was imprisoned for two years, the marquis survived the massacre and even recovered his estate, eventually living to a ripe old age.

MESMERISM AND SPIRITUALISM IN THE UNITED STATES

You may be wondering by now, why I have devoted so much space to the rise of mesmerism. The answer lies in the fact that the movement underwent a strange transformation when it spread to the United States. The mesmeric movement in Europe had been a scientific revolution. Mesmeric techniques were medical procedures, bogus or not, for healing the sick. But it was the spiritual side of the practice that caught on in the New World. The spiritually hungry American public saw in mesmerism not a medical breakthrough, but a religious power. Could the mesmeric state, for example, be employed to establish contact with some spiritual realm?

This spiritualization of mesmerism gave rise to new cults and sects fascinated by the interrelationships between spiritual and physical health. These two aspects of everyday life were considered totally interrelated by these groups. Whole religions and even some contemporary medical movements stem from this original spiritualization of Mesmer's discoveries, real or imaginary. Some of the people interviewed later in this book, such as Louise Hay and Dr. Janet Quinn, come or work from these traditions. So it is essential to understand these historical connections in order to comprehend the metaphysical undercurrents behind these interviews. These same undercurrents gave rise, in part, to the human potentials movement of the 1960s and 1970s, which was the immediate progenitor of today's holistic health revolution.

20   The story of mesmerism's exodus from science to religion has been chronicled by Dr. Robert C. Fuller in his books *Mesmerism and the American Cure of Souls* and *Alternative Medicine and American Religious Life*. Dr. Fuller is Professor of Philosophy and Religious Studies at Bradley University in Peoria, Illinois. Much of the following discussion is based on these sources.

Mesmerism was introduced into the United States by Charles Poyen, a former French medical student who toured New England in 1838. He had learned magnetism while visiting the West Indies, where the plantation owners often experimented with the phenomenon on their slaves. Unlike his confreres in Europe, the enterprising Frenchman offered stage demonstrations of his skills to America's eager public, from whom he drew clients for private instruction. It is said that Poyen was neither physically comely nor particularly charismatic, but his obvious earnestness and the pure novelty of his claims guaranteed his success.

A second factor that prompted the success of the mesmeric movement in the United States was Poyen's discovery of Cynthia Gleason, who became clairvoyant when entranced. She was not well-educated and had been a textile worker, but while magnetized, she could diagnose the physical problems of people brought to her or even those in distant locations. She also exhibited most of the standard phenomena of mesmerism, including the somnambulistic trance, insensitivity to pin pricks and so forth. For his general stage performances, Poyen would lecture on mesmerism, entrance Cynthia, and then invite the public to come to the stage and pinch, prick, or otherwise experiment with her. Demonstrations of her powers of second sight were usually restricted to medical students or physicians, however.

Mr. Poyen traveled with Cynthia Gleason for several months, wrote a book on his experiences and then returned to France. Miss Gleason thereupon left the public limelight and returned to her previous work.

Even though the French magnetist's tour was relatively short, mesmerism caught on in the New World and soon several other practitioners were demonstrating the phenomenon. Lectures and public demonstrations of mesmerism became, in fact, a popular form of public entertainment. It was during this time that mesmerism underwent that strange odyssey from science to religion.

The consensus of the mesmerists was that if a subject were to be entranced deeply enough, he or she could be freed from any reliance on the five senses—thereby placing him or her in direct contact with the spiritual realms. Entering into a direct relationship with the cosmos became mesmerism's ultimate promise. Mesmerized subjects would be asked to establish contact with these realms and describe them, or even relate messages from their denizens. Experiments to establish contact with the dead were even conducted, a practice which had been explored in Europe, but without much popularity. Because of these strange proceedings, mesmerism gradually lost its identity as a healing procedure and became a method for exploring the inner world of consciousness.

In commenting on this model, Dr. Robert C. Fuller writes in his *Alternative Medicine and American Religious Life* that "The mesmerists' psychological continuum defined both an experiential path initiated by the healing process and a metaphysical hierarchy. That is, the 'deeper' levels of consciousness achieved during the mesmerizing process put individuals into contact with qualitatively 'higher' planes of reality. The mesmerists were thus articulating a healing philosophy that attributed the true cause of healing and personal growth to a distinctively metaphysical, as opposed to physiological or psychological, agent."

Such a metaphysical doctrine was bound to be popular to the New England public of the 1840s. This part of the country was famous for its spiritual unrest and eventually served as the breeding grounds for several novel religious movements. The rise of the Industrial Revolution, the decline of religious literalism, and the fact that the population was a melting pot of immigrants from diverse cultural backgrounds contributed to this unrest. It seemed as though the New Englanders, having left their previous social and religious identities behind them, were searching for a replacement.

In this respect, mesmerism offered not only a method for interacting with the higher realms, but a complete religious philosophy. Some of the mesmerists even copied the stage setting of religious revivalism by traveling lecture circuits, preaching that people could overcome their infirmities by entering into higher consciousness. Physical health was contingent on spiritual health. If people could live their lives in concordance with the cosmic order, they would be imbued with nature's own life force and reap its benefits. Being healed of a physical problem is not due to magnetism itself, but results from contact with cosmic forces.

With the development of this doctrine came the original basis of holistic thinking: that "good health" results from living in complete

22 harmony with the universe. This fundamental insight became the underlying principle behind several new medical and religious movements that were to follow... some of them still extant today.

The mesmeric movement lasted through the 1840s before it declined and evaporated from the cultural scene. The reasons for its demise are a matter of conjecture. Probably the main reason, which isn't emphasized by Fuller, was the rise of popular Spiritualism in the late 1840s. This new religion was founded by three sisters in upper New York state, whose family home had been plagued by a poltergeist. The phenomena consisted chiefly of mysterious rappings in the house, day and night. Two of the sisters, Kate and Margaret Fox, learned that they could communicate with the "ghost" through a code. That the spirit world could be contacted through such raps or through table-turning caught on like wildfire. (Such claims made excellent copy for the popular press, which no doubt expedited the spread of the religion.) Soon people came forth who claimed that they could establish direct contact with the dead while entranced, and such individuals became the first "sensitives" or "mediums."

The exact manner by which the rise of Spiritualism contributed to the decline of mesmerism is rather simple. To begin with, it became a new fad that replaced the public's interest in mesmerism. But more importantly, it pulled the rug from under the mesmerists' feet. Remember that they were dependent upon finding exceptionally good subjects for their stage demonstrations. Some experts have suggested that these subjects either left the stage or were drawn to Spiritualism to become the first public psychics—giving public demonstrations of their powers or bringing through "lectures" from the spirit world. (The current practice of channeling is, in fact, merely a reprise of this earlier practice and relies upon the same phenomenon—i.e., that dissociation is a common psychological phenomenon and skill.) This switch from mesmerism to 'Spiritualism is exemplified, for instance, in the life and career of Andrew Jackson Davis (1826–1910), the Poughkeepsie Seer. He discovered that he was an exceptional mesmeric subject while experimenting with a local tailor in New York City. Whole books on metaphysical subjects were dictated by the entranced subject, and these books became immensely popular in their day. But while Davis never claimed that these works were dictated by spirit intelligences, later in life he claimed to see spirits of the dead and to be sensitive to their world.

Eventually he left the employment of the mesmerists and worked on his own.

Because of the exodus of the best magnetic subjects to Spiritualism (where they could play center stage), the mesmeric movement declined and died. But its center philosophy that our health and prosperity result from living in harmony with the universe remained popular. It exerted a formidable power in American culture and, as pointed out earlier, considerably influenced nineteenth century medicine. Metaphysical factors were present in hydropathy (the formal name for "water cures") and homeopathy, both founded on the principle that there were basic interrelationships between the spiritual and material worlds. The founder of homeopathy, German physician Samuel Hahnemann, believed that small doses of drugs work spiritually on the body's vital forces. Two other medical movements from these years still popular today—chiropractics and osteopathic medicine—were built upon this fundamental belief. Each of these two disciplines will be briefly examined.

Chiropractics was the brainchild of Daniel David Palmer (1845–1913), who began his career as a grocer in Iowa. Even though he had never received much of a formal education, he read widely and was fascinated by philosophy and metaphysics. Soon he was experimenting with mesmerism, during which he learned that rubbing and slapping the body was a crucial factor in magnetic healing. He felt that this discovery explained an incident from his earlier life: Once when his mother was in extreme pain, he had cured her by placing his hands on her head.

D. D. Palmer soon gave up his grocery business, became a magnetic healer, and enjoyed a successful practice for nine years. There is some evidence that he was a gifted clairvoyant, for he could diagnose a client's problem on sight and sometimes took on their symptoms.

The science of chiropractics was born when Palmer was trying to heal a deaf janitor, whose problem stemmed from a work-related back injury. (Of course, the strange connection between a back problem and deafness suggests that the disorder was functional and not organic.) While magnetizing his back by manipulating the vertebrae, the patient's hearing returned. The surprised healer next tried the same procedure on a second patient and found that manipulating the spine, in general, had curative powers. The reason, he suggested, was that health is based on a life force in the body which can be blocked by

24 spinal problems. Manipulating the backbone to release this vital energy should be the physician's fundamental responsibility. The role that cosmology played in early chiropractics is no better illustrated than in Palmer's own book *The Chiropractor's Adjustor,* which expounds philosophy as frequently as medicine. The fundamental law of chiropractics, he wrote, is that physical life is the reflection of a divine reality. This metaphysical reality is channeled into mankind through a vital energy, which is essential to life's maintenance. It is with this force that the chiropractor works. Palmer went even further by proposing that each of us is "but an epitome" of the universe, a microcosmic reflection of the cosmic order.

Chiropractic medicine was further promoted by D. D. Palmer's son, who also emphasized that the practice should not be separated from the metaphysics behind it.

Osteopathic medicine was founded by the son of a Virginia minister. Andrew Taylor Still (1828–1917) received his education through home instruction which included some medicine. (Like many ministers of that era, his father was a self-taught physician of sorts.) It could be said that religion and healing were combined in his mind from childhood. Still worked with his father when the family moved to the Midwest, where they often ministered to the indigenous Indians. These communities were periodically struck by severe epidemics and Still soon learned basic physiology, diagnosis, clinical pharmacology, and simple surgical procedures. But medicine in those days was crude and unreliable, and Still was often frustrated by the capricious results of his ministrations. His rejection of conventional medicine was finalized later in life, when he sat by helplessly as his three children died from spinal meningitis.

Since he was by nature a religious man, Still began to theorize that there must be some sort of medical practice that placed mankind in harmony with God, thereby curing physical illness. He subsequently set himself up as a healer specializing in drugless medicine. Working from the mesmeric concept of a subtle fluid in the body, Still based his practice on shaking and otherwise manipulating the body. His practice wasn't too popular and he was even forced to move to a different city!

Andrew Taylor Still's interest in manipulating the body included bone setting, which was part and parcel of conventional nineteenth century medicine. The self-made doctor soon discovered, however, that setting and manipulating bones often cured unrelated problems his patients were suffering. Osteopathic medicine was born when he successfully healed the son of a United States senator, whose cardiac problem was then untreatable by conventional medicine. While the cures he implemented were based on physically manipulating the body, the guiding force of his work was letting "the highest of force" from God balance itself in the body to create perfect health. It was the old magnetic philosophy revamped into a new and more contemporary form.

Both chiropractics and osteopathic medicine survive to this day and enjoy the official sanction of established medicine. The long story behind the emergence of these practices into the mainstream won't be summarized in this chapter. (Some of this history is given in Dr. Robert C. Fuller's *Alternative Medicine and American Religious Life.*) Suffice to say that, over the years, the procedures of the chiropractors and osteopathic practioners became divorced from their metaphysical foundations. Both of these medical practices were eventually secularized, and, slowly but surely, they won the respect of the medical community—which saw the importance of their tools, if not their philosophy. Today, osteopathic medicine is so integrated into the Western medical establishment that a D.O. has the same legal and professional rights as an M.D., while chiropractors recently won hospital priviledges in California. But lost is the fact that such practices were meant to bring people into better harmony with God and the universe.

There was a third religious/medical movement that emerged from the mid-nineteenth century that also remains popular today, but this school of thought has retained its metaphysical emphasis. This movement is called New Thought and served as the basis for the rise of Christian Science and, sometime later, the Church of Religious Science and its "Science of Mind" philosophy. So for the remainder of this chapter, the history of New Thought philosophy will be outlined, with an emphasis on its contribution to contemporary issues in religion, health and, personal growth.

NEW THOUGHT AND ITS LEGACY

The spiritual and medical movements outlined in the previous section were based on theories dating back to early mesmerism. Each posited the existence of a life force connecting us with the cosmos.

26 That recovery from illness is contingent upon balancing this force within the body was correlated with such thinking.

Aside from chiropractics, magnetism, and homeopathy came the emergence of New Thought philosophy. The central message of this system wasn't that subtle energies caused remarkable cures, but that health and healing were the result of right *thinking*. Maintaining the correct thoughts and directing them toward some cosmic "source" would, by itself, produce beneficial results—both spiritual and material. One metaphor found throughout early New Thought literature was that the mind is a daguerreotype (photograph) of the universe. It therefore followed that the cosmic order would respond to changes in a person's thoughts. The popular concept of the "power of positive thinking" is, in fact, central to New Thought and was coined by the movement's promoters.

This type of metaphysics is so firmly ingrained into today's popular culture that few people realize that it isn't merely folk wisdom, but a carefully crafted spiritual philosophy with origins in the nineteenth century. So to understand the basis of this philosophy, let's travel back in time to February 16, 1802, to Lebanon, New Hampshire. That was the date and birthplace of Phineas P. Quimby, later to become one of the most fascinating personalities ever to emerge from American religion.

Born the son of a blacksmith, Phineas P. Quimby moved to Belfast, Maine, in early life. He began his working career making clocks, but took an interest in medicine when he contracted tuberculosis. He was treated with the worthless drugs of his day, which he felt completely poisoned his body. He had given up hope for recovery when his disease spontaneously and inexplicably remitted. The next crucial point in his life came in 1836 when he witnessed a stage demonstration of mesmerism. Intrigued by the performance, he began experimenting on his own and soon discovered his first exceptional subject. We don't know much about Lucius Burkman, other than that he became powerfully psychic when mesmerized and could diagnose and prescribe herbal remedies for his clients.

It was while engaged in this work that Quimby began to suspect that their cures were based on more than insight, magnetism, and herbs. Sometimes his clients recovered upon taking ineffective or worthless remedies prescribed by Burkman, and the implications of such observations were not lost on the experimenter. Quimby was similarly puzzled when, during one personal session, Burkman diagnosed his employer with a kidney problem—which the healer previously suspected. The mesmerized subject treated him with the laying on of hands and the pain promptly disappeared. But the cure left Quimby thinking: Was he really cured of his kidney problem, or had he been mistaken in thinking the organ was diseased? Was it possible that the pain vanished because he *expected* it to. Was the mind, in fact, the key player in health rather than some mesmeric force?

Phineas Quimby was drawn more and more to this line of thinking as he continued experimenting both with Burkman and with clairvoyance in general. Eventually he, too, developed the sixth sense and began diagnosing clients on sight. This research led the healer to experiment with procedures for purely mental healing. Such healing practices, he posited, should be based on religious belief and right thinking, thereby bypassing the cumbersome use of mesmerism. The clockmaker-turned-physician eventually set up practice as an unorthodox practitioner in Portland, Maine, in 1859. The premise of his practice was that recovery from sickness came through changes in thought processes; that disease is, in fact, the product of mistaken beliefs. Simplified to its basic tenet, the key to the system was that a sick person could overcome his or her infirmities by correcting *belief* in disease.

Writing in a popular magazine in 1859, Quimby explained that "The trouble is in the mind, for the body is only the house for the mind to dwell in.... Therefore, if your mind has been deceived by some invisible enemy you have put into it the form of a disease, with or without your knowledge. By my theory or truth, I come in contact with your enemy, and restore you to health and happiness. This I do partly mentally, and partly by talking till I correct the wrong impression and establish the Truth, and the Truth is the cure."

Perhaps this kind of thinking was simplistic, but it would later serve as the foundation for psychoneuroimmunology... not that disease *is* a faulty belief, but that psychological factors (or patterns of thought) can contribute to the disease process.

Even epidemics could be explained as the result of faulty belief systems. Smallpox, explained the Maine healer, only existed because the current medical and religious establishments promoted its dangers and brainwashed society in general. Left out of the explanation, of course, was where smallpox came from to begin with.

28   Working from within this framework, what specific procedures could the healer employ to treat the sick? The procedures Phineas Quimby used for mental healing were prescribed by the patient's physical location. If he or she were living in some distant city, Quimby would "correct" the patient's problems for a small fee by correspondence. The healer took a more dynamic approach to those patients who came to see him. Since healing takes place with the mind, it really wasn't necessary to explain much to the patient. Because of his experience with diagnostic clairvoyance, Quimby knew that he could communicate with his patients on a purely unspoken plane. So he would sit with his patients, diagnose their problems through clairvoyance, and then "explain" the mistaken beliefs underlying them. He would then use the power of the mind to impress new beliefs onto the client's psyche, thereby curing him or her. Sometimes body manipulation was included in order to intensify these communications.

This form of mental healing could even be practiced over long distances, since the psyche was not constrained by geographical restrictions. Entering into the thought processes of a person in some distant community presented little problem.

It may strike the reader that these practices lacked spirituality, since their emphasis was the power of the healer or the mind. But this would be a mistaken interpretation of Phineas Quimby's metaphysical system. He stressed in his writings that the healing power comes from some spiritual realm. Cures take place because mental healing works on the spiritual side of matter, from which physical matter is a mere reflection.

Unlike many unorthodox practitioners of his era, Quimby was openly critical of both priests and physicians. He felt that they had seriously contributed to society's mistaken beliefs in disease, but he remained religious in his personal life and believed in a loving but impersonal God.

In short, Phineas P. Quimby set the foundations for New Thought philosophy through his writings and his doctrines. When he died in 1866, he left behind a legacy that would permanently change American religion. Much of this change came not from the healer himself, but from those he cured, who became the first spokespeople for New Thought's spiritual message. Three of these people particularly spread this form of popular metaphysics: Warren Felt Evans,

Julius A. Dresser, and Mary Baker Patterson (later Eddy) were patient's of Phineas P. Quimby toward the end of his life. Evans (1817–1889) popularized New Thought philosophy not by founding a religious movement, but by writing books for the general public introducing such concepts. Even though he set up practice as a healer, he is best remembered today for books such as *The Divine Law of Cure* and *The Primitive Mind Cure* published in the 1880s.

Julius A. Dresser (1838– ?) collaborated with his wife Annetta G. Seabury in setting up practice as a healer in Boston in 1882, where he popularized New Thought philosophy. Their work was carried on by their son Horatio through his many books on religion, philosophy, and psychology. (A complete and engaging history of the New Thought movement, which includes lengthy chapters on these figures, can be found in Dr. Charles S. Braden's *Spirits in Rebellion: The Rise and Development of New Thought.)*

It is unfortunate that, today, people such as Warren Felt Evans and Julius Dresser remain historical curiosities. They had no personal influence on popular religious culture. The same cannot be said, however, of the famous (or perhaps infamous) Mary Baker Eddy (1821–1910). A neurotic and difficult woman, Mrs. Eddy combined her former mentor's teachings with her own forceful personality to form her own religious movement, Christian Science, still popular and influential in contemporary United States.

Mary Baker Eddy was born on July 16, 1821, and received a conservative Calvinist upbringing in New Hampshire. She was given her formal education at home since her frequent illnesses kept her from public school. These endless problems were undoubtedly psychological in nature, and most of her biographers refer to them simply as nervous disorders. The future Mrs. Eddy married George Washington Glover when she was twenty-two years old and the couple moved to South Carolina, but her husband's death from yellow fever left her a widow with a posthumously born child to rear. Her previous nervous problems returned, confining her to bed, where she would request people to cradle and rock her... perhaps an early indication of her lifelong pattern of extreme dependence on her friends and coworkers.

The future founder of Christian Science displayed a second habit during these years upon which her detractors later seized. She began living in the homes of her relatives, often to their regret, since she would invariably make considerable demands on them.

30   Mrs. Eddy was later married to Daniel Patterson in 1853, a traveling dentist from New Hampshire, but she remained bedridden for
most of their relationship.

Since her health problems wouldn't respond to conventional
medicine, Mary Baker (Patterson) began searching for unorthodox
cures. It was apparently her husband who directed her to Phineas P.
Quimby, then practicing mind cures in Portland, Maine. Mr.
Patterson originally wrote to him in 1861, requesting his help in
restoring his wife's health. Mary made the trip to Maine by herself
sometime later. Through their sessions together, Quimby "cured" his
new patient, who took up the cause of mental healing with both grati-
tude and enthusiasm. That she was restored to health wasn't surprising, since her lifelong infirmity was probably hysterical in nature.
But the maintenance of her health was probably due to the raw energy she threw into her rescuer's cause. Mrs. Patterson's commitment to
the science of mental healing was reconfirmed in 1866 when she fell
on some frosty pavement and was knocked unconscious. She later
claimed (without support) that her physician pronounced her permanently crippled, but she rallied and recovered through the lessons
she had learned in Maine.

In point of fact, Mary Baker Patterson was *forced* to cure herself,
for her mentor had recently died. Frank Podmore, a British student of
the paranormal, wrote in 1909 in his book *From Mesmer to Christian
Science* (originally published under the title *Mesmerism and Christian
Science)* that "Mrs. Eddy was forced to fight the illness and depression resulting from the accident with her own right hand, even if the
weapon which brought victory had been forged by another." He cau-
tioned his readers, however, that even though she recovered, "... in
fact, as we learn from the affidavit of the doctor who attended her, her
injury was not of a severe character." Some experts on the history of
religion believe that Christian Science, as a sect, dates from this
episode.

Despite the inconsequential nature of the injury, it is clear that
Mrs. Patterson saw in her cure the foundation for her life's work. She
soon began proselytizing for the cause of mental healing. She first
flirted briefly with Spiritualism, but later set herself up as a mental
healer, teaching from the manuscripts of Phineas P. Quimby. Over the
subsequent years, however, her emphasis slowly began to change.

When she returned to Lynn, Massachusetts, in 1870, she brought
with her a young student and set up shop as a metaphysical teacher
and healer. She remained in the city for the next eleven years, during
which she began work on her *Science and Health with Key to the
Scriptures.* She also married for the third time, on this occasion to
Gilbert A. Eddy, a successful sewing machine salesman. (Mrs. Eddy
was fifty-six years old by this time, but she claimed to be forty. She
had divorced Daniel Patterson for desertion some time earlier.) While
composing her grand opus, Mrs. Eddy took Phineas P. Quimby's philosophy and presented it as her own. She later even claimed no
indebtedness to her former mentor or his theories.

Even to this day, official spokespeople for the Church of Christ,
Scientist claim that she merely employed the Quimby manuscripts as
stepping stones to her own philosophy. Such is probably not the case.
By objectively reading both the collected writings of Phineas Quimby
and Mrs. Eddy, it is clear that they present the exact same views and
doctrines. Mrs. Eddy even borrowed her former teacher's idiosyncratic style of capitalizing key words—sometimes the same words—in
her writings. (These facts are not disputed by historical scholars. The
manner by which she drew upon Phineas P. Quimby, even down to
small particulars, is discussed by Dr. Julius Silberger in his book
*Mary Baker Eddy: An Interpretive Biography of the Founder of
Christian Science.*)

Even the real authorship of *Science and Health* is disputable. It is
certain that Mary Baker Eddy drafted the manuscript, but the book
was unreadable and was edited and rewritten by the Rev. James
Henry Wiggin, who understood the project purely as an editorial
chore. The Rev. Wiggin was a Unitarian minister and he even inserted one of his sermons into the text!

The fact that her philosophy was borrowed from a progenitor mat-
tered little to the New England public. Mrs. Eddy's classes prospered
and she eventually became a relatively wealthy woman. She officially
founded the Church of Christ (Science) in Boston in 1879. Mrs.
Eddy's simple message that healing could take place through the
power of the mind was so popular that thirty thousand people sought
entry to the church. Services for the congregations included prayer,
readings from the Bible and *Science and Health,* and a talk by Mrs.
Eddy herself.

32   From these populist beginnings, Christian Science and its creed spread from state to state and permanently established itself in the United States. The denomination's primary theology is that God is everything and equitable with Mind, thereby demonstrating that matter and disease have no real existence. Mrs. Eddy explains this creed herself in *Science and Health,* where she states that "Christian Science explains all cause and effect as mental, not physical. It lifts the veil of mystery from Soul and body. It shows the scientific relation of man to God, disentangles the interlaced ambiguities of being, and sets free the imprisoned thought. In divine Science, the universe, including man, is spiritual, harmonious and eternal. Science shows that what is termed *matter* is but the subjective state of what is termed by the author mortal mind."

Because of this philosophy, church members in principle refuse to let physicians treat sickness or disease. Sickness, it is taught, can be overcome by changes in thinking and Christian Science practitioners should be brought in if prayer falters. Or such practitioners can employ methods similar to those originally pioneered by Phineas P. Quimby.

Whether or not such practices result in the permanent cure of serious disease is a fascinating controversy in science and religion. Most forms of unorthodox medicine claim their fair share of cures. Christian Science is no different in this respect, and books continue to be written on remarkable remissions reported by church members. *

Mrs. Eddy's life subsequent to the rise of her church is steeped in intrigue and controversy. She was involved in several bitter disputes with former students and her own church officials, and became close to paranoid in her later years. Probably the most bizarre episode in her life dates from her last illness in Boston. She was so concerned with her public image that she hired an impersonator to ride the streets in her carriage to prove to the faithful that she was still in perfect health. Secretly, though, she was dying and sending for dentists and doctors to ease her suffering. She died of pneumonia on December 3, 1910, reportedly dependent on morphine. Her last wish was that her disciples should claim she died from "mental murder" and not from natural causes.

* The most recent of these is *Spiritual Healing in a Scientific Age* by Robert Peel (New York: Harper and Row, 1987). This book is written from a strongly sectarian position and probably will not impress more critical readers.

The fact that Mrs. Eddy was so eccentric and difficult in her personal life is irrelevant to the message of her philosophy. The most notable characteristic of her religion, on the other hand, is its extremity. Since its followers do not believe in *the reality of disease,* they often refuse treatment. Robert Peel explains in his book *Spiritual Healing in a Scientific Age* that when stricken with illness, the Christian Scientist must place his/her faith in medicine or faith, but not in both. (Of course, such a position is complicated when children are involved. Despite our constitutional rights to freedom of religion, the United States courts have not been sympathetic to parents whose children suffered or died because of these beliefs. Manslaughter convictions have been given in such cases. Whether these court decisions will be upheld should constitute a fascinating future chapter in American jurisprudence.)

Even though Christian Science represents New Thought philosophy in its most fundamental form, it is not the only religious tradition that emerged from Phineas Quimby's original insight. Several related movements claiming New Thought legacy were born in the late nineteenth century. So many separate groups came into existence, in fact, that national conferences on New Thought philosophy were organized in the late 1890s. Included in these groups were the Unity School of Christianity (founded in 1890 by Charles and Myrtle Fillmore), Divine Science (created in the 1880s by Kentucky-born healer Nona L. Brooks), and (sometime later) Religious Science. While most of these groups had limited followings, Religious Science eventually became extremely successful. Since some of the interviews in this book reflect this spiritual tradition, its history and chief philosophy will be briefly outlined.

The founder of the movement was Ernest Holmes, who never expected his insights to be institutionalized into a formal religion. Perhaps it was prophetic that, like Phineas P. Quimby, he was born into a poor family in Maine on January 21, 1887. The family's limited financial resources prevented him from receiving much formal education, but Holmes was intellectually inclined and read voraciously. Intellectual pursuits must have been a family trait, for his brother, Fenwicke, procured a college education and became a Congregationalist minister in California. Ernest Holmes eventually trekked west and worked for his brother's church, but was sidetracked when he chanced on the writings of Swami Ramacharaka (the

34   pen name of the British yogi W. W. Atkinson). These popular works introduced him to Eastern philosophy. The future spiritual leader gradually began integrating Eastern spirituality with the writings of such New Thought leaders as Mary Baker Eddy, Christian D. Larson, and others. A third crucial influence in Holmes's spiritual evolution were the books of Thomas Troward (1844–1916), a British philosopher and judge whose writings reflected his interest in psychology of the unconscious. Troward had lived in India and was instrumental in introducing Western readers to that country's spiritual heritage.

Ernest Holmes's personal philosophy was a synthesis of popular psychology and New Thought philosophy, liberally dowsed with concepts borrowed from the East. Sometime in 1917, he and his brother, Fenwicke, founded a metaphysical institute in California to promote these teachings. They undertook to publish a New Thought magazine in 1919. They also lectured widely in Los Angeles and Long Beach before undertaking speaking tours on the East Coast. It is important to note, however, that the Holmeses presented their philosophy as a metaphysical system and not as a religion.

The next phase in the development of Religious Science came when Ernest Holmes read the works of Emma Curtis Hopkins, a former student of Mrs. Eddy's and a mystic in her own right. She taught privately in Chicago, where she had earlier founded the Christian Science Theological Seminary in 1887. Dr. Charles Braden described Holmes's meeting with his elderly mentor in his book *Spirits in Rebellion: The Rise and Development of New Thought:*

> Though well along in years, she was still teaching, at least individuals. He sought her out and was ushered into her presence. She was always the grand lady, formally dressed and wearing a hat as though about to go out. She greeted him coolly and began to talk. She talked steadily for an hour, and then he knew he had had his first lesson. He returned again and again. She eventually unbent and they became fast friends. His association with her added a new dimension to his thinking. He was to rate her along with Eckhart as the greatest of the mystics. It was not, says Fenwicke, through this experience that he had his first intimation of "cosmic consciousness" but here it became a basic element of religion to him.

The climax to Ernest Holmes's career came in 1926 when he combined psychology, mysticism, and New Thought philosophy to write his ever popular book the *Science of Mind*. The volume was designed as a textbook for students of his teachings. The metaphysical system outlined in the book speaks of an ineffable mind behind the universe, to which we are connected on some unconscious level. Tapping into this channel promises to unleash our creative forces. The fruits of such a relationship are health, happiness, and a prosperous life.

Critics of New Thought philosophy have specifically condemned the suggestion that prosperity should be related to spiritual development. More conventional theologians often have faulted the United Church of Religious Science, particularly, for its "prosperity consciousness"—i.e., that members of the church should use religion in the search for material reward. This is really misrepresenting what I think Ernest Holmes and his followers were trying to say. I think the message in New Thought and Religious Science is that material benefits are side effects of the search for spiritual satisfaction in life.

As pointed out earlier, Holmes resisted calling his philosophy a religion, but his followers wanted to organize and the Institute of Religious Science and Philosophy was founded in Los Angeles in 1927. The Institute laid the foundation for Religious Science to incorporate into a formal church. *Science of Mind* magazine began publishing that same year, which remains today the official organ of the United Church of Religious Science. The church is still headquartered on Sixth Street and New Hampshire Street near the building they originally took over in 1937. Ernest Holmes himself lived the rest of his life in a beautiful two-story home on Los Feliz Boulevard, which is still the epitome of Los Angeles ritz. (I visited the house in the late 1960s when the current owners hosted a get-together for people interested in parapsychology. I found it extremely impressive!)

It could be said that Holmes enjoyed the fruits of his philosophy, including relative happiness and enviable prosperity. But he never believed that his philosophy was some final revelation and never blessed the institutionalization of his metaphysics. (A leading figure in the church once told me that Holmes invariably referred to the Sixth Street building as "the ediface" and not a church!) He died a wealthy man in 1960, and the United Church of Religious Science currently represents New Thought philosophy in its most successful and popular form.

36 So what is the true nature of spiritual and physical healing? Is recovery from disease merely the workings of the body's incredibly complex immune system... sometimes helped by its connections with the brain and endocrine system? Or does recovery from serious illness come when we tap into the universe's cosmic life force? Or does right thinking create perfect wellness by virtue of the reflective nature of the cosmos?

I couldn't even begin to resolve such issues. Maybe each of these possibilities is true in some instances. This lengthy introduction has served merely to introduce these concepts. They will be explored in greater depth during the course of the following interviews and chapters. In this respect, I certainly hope this book will not be considered the final say on these matters, but as an embarking point for each reader's growth and self-discovery.

ABOUT THE
INTERVIEWS

Early in 1986 I received a letter from the staff of *Science of Mind* magazine inviting me to contribute feature interviews to them. This periodical is the official organ of the United Church of Religious Science and is published in Los Angeles, where I live. Mr. John Niendorf, the editor, explained that I could choose the people with whom I wished to speak. While they didn't have to come specifically from a Religious Science background, they had to reflect the essential message of Science of Mind philosophy—better living through better psychological and spiritual health.

I am not nor ever have been a member of the United Church of Religious Science. I was invited to contribute to the magazine because of my experience writing on psychology and parapsychology.

The eleven interviews published in this book are reprinted from *Science of Mind* magazine, where they appeared between 1986 and 1989. I especially chose people researching either the powers of the mind or the relationship between psychology and spirituality. One or two were suggested to me by Mr. Niendorf. After I familiarized myself with the work of my prospective guest, I prepared a blueprint, consisting of several questions for the interview. I then submitted these to Mr. Niendorf for his input. We worked enjoyably and constructively together until changes in the church's editorial division led him to leave the magazine. I continued on briefly under the new editor before deciding to focus my efforts elsewhere.

The interviews that follow are reprinted exactly as they were published in *Science of Mind*. On rare occasion, however, I have redraft-

38 ed my comments in order to delete specific reference to Religious Science. These remarks have been slightly rewritten in more generic form to insure a wider readership. The exception to this rule is the interview with Louise L. Hay. Since she comes specifically from a Religious Science background, that emphasis had to be retained. No changes whatsoever have been made in the responses. The original tape-recorded interviews were heavily edited for better language use and expression, but each participant read over his or her contribution before we committed to press.

I have refrained from presenting these interviews in the order they were originally published. They correspond instead to the order of the topics introduced in the Introduction. The first part of the book is devoted to the interrelationship between the mind and the body. Part II explores the nature of spiritual healing, while Part III consists of three interviews on religious healing and personal growth. Included with each interview is a short biography of my guest, followed by some remarks on the settings for the talks—which were conducted everywhere from busy airports to my living room! To break up the interviews, I have inserted two profiles of people I've met in my career whose work contributes to the book's scope. These profiles seemed to weave naturally into the formal interviews and complement them.

I hope that you enjoy reading these talks as much as I delighted in conducting them. Working with *Science of Mind* gave me the opportunity to meet several fascinating people and conducting these interviews certainly added to my own personal growth. I feel privileged to share them with you.

PART I. WAYS TO BETTER LIVING

1 OVERCOMING STRESS IN THE WORKPLACE

AN INTERVIEW WITH
KENNETH R. PELLETIER, PH.D.

B I O G R A P H Y

Kenneth R. Pelletier received his Ph.D. from the University of California, Berkeley, and an honorary M.D. for his work in international health care. He also studied at the C. G. Jung Institute in Zurich, Switzerland. He is currently an associate clinical professor at the University of California School of Medicine, San Francisco, and is senior consultant with United States Corporate Health Management in Santa Monica. Dr. Pelletier serves as advisor to the United States Department of Health and Human Services, the National Institute of Mental Health, Blue Cross, the Canadian Ministry of Health, and the World Health Organization. He is the author of several books, including the best-selling *Mind As Healer Mind As Slayer*, as well as *Toward a Science of Consciousness, Holistic Medicine: From Stress to Optimum Health*, and *Longevity: Fulfilling our Biological Potential*. His most recent book is *Healthy People in Unhealthy Places: Stress and Fitness at Work*. He is currently a resident of Alamo, California.

The chance to sit down and talk with Dr. Kenneth Pelletier was a rare opportunity, for he is one of the true "superstars" of the contemporary health movement. Such terms as "holistic health," "mind over body," and "psychosomatic" have become catchwords in popular culture. But it was Dr. Pelletier and others who first devoted their careers to showing the intricate ways that the mind contributes to both health and illness. His book *Mind As Healer Mind As Slayer* is a classic in the field of psychoneuroimmunology.

The setting for this interview was Dr. Pelletier's wonderful custom home in the hills on the west side of the San Francisco Bay. It was set in one of the most bucolic scenes imaginable, so I could hardly believe it when my host said he was moving. Dr. Pelletier seemed to enjoy our talk, too, since—he said dolorously—it is rare for interviewers to read his books! The psychologist's interests have veered a bit since *Mind As Healer Mind As Slayer* was published in 1977. Environmental and work stresses can interact with purely psychological determinates of health and that was the subject of the interview.

D. Scott Rogo: Dr. Pelletier, do you believe that psychological factors, or what we call "the mind," can make a person physically ill?

Kenneth R. Pelletier: I don't think there's any doubt about it. Psychological factors—stress in particular—are being increasingly recognized as a major contributing factor in what we often see as chronic degenerative disease. By this, I mean such conditions as heart disease, depressive conditions, arthritis, and cancer. This last possibility remains controversial, but stress certainly contributes to cancer. Chronic lung problems, muscular problems, and lower back pain can also be included. Not that stress is, in itself, the only factor.

But it is probably the major contributing factor to what we see. *43*
There's a vast range of disorders which we can refer to as psychophys-
ical, psychosomatic, or life-style related, and stress plays a major role
in them all, according to the new area of psychoneuroimmunology.

**Do you consider stress to be the primary psychological
health hazard in the United States today?**

It probably is. Taken together, stress and depression—and depression is frequently a reaction to excessive stress—represent our two
major psychological hazards. They, in turn, often lead to the development of physical problems, though they can remain disorders in
themselves.

How does stress affect the body physiologically?

First, I think it is important to point out that the popular literature
makes a big mistake when it says all stress is uniformly destructive.
That's definitely not the case. What's critical is how we respond to
stress. I also think it is important to understand that there are two
basic kinds of stress, which I call Type 1 and Type 2 stressors.

What are the differences between these two kinds of stressors?

The first type is what I refer to in my book *Mind As Healer Mind
As Slayer* as a Type 1 stress response. It is not destructive, and it
occurs under a very particular set of circumstances. It occurs when
the stress is immediate, identifiable, and resolvable. Try to remember
a time when you perceived that your life was in danger. It might have
been when the airplane you were in bounced on the runway too many
times, or when there was a jolt in the air, or when a car swerved into
your lane while you were driving on the freeway. Think about what
happens in these situations. To begin with there's a tremendous state
of arousal. You move the wheel of the car very quickly and your
response time is extraordinary. You start to breathe rapidly and shal-
lowly. And then, usually when the event is over, you let out a sigh of
relief. This sigh is a signal from the mind to the body saying that
everything is okay. You can then begin to breathe more deeply from
the abdomen, and you begin to fill the lungs completely.

The point I'm making is that under these special conditions you
are roused to meet a specific demand. Certain electrical changes
occur in the brain, biochemical changes occur in the body, and phys-

44   iological alterations take place in the organ systems of the body. Then after meeting the challenge, your body enters a period of relaxation.

How does this period of relaxation manifest?

We tremble a little bit. We feel weak and a little disoriented and shaky. We might notice that we are starting to sweat, whereas we weren't sweating before. This shaky, disoriented period is actually beneficial since it compensates for the prior peak response. We need this compensatory period, this rebound, and it seems to occur in every cell of the body. Now although the response isn't pleasant, this Type 1 stress response is entirely beneficial. In fact, we'd be dead if we didn't have it. For example, you'd step out in the street, a car would come toward you, and you'd just stand there! The result would be an accident. This form of stress is a biologically adaptive response we've had since we first evolved as a species. It's been called the "fight or flight" response. It is very primitive and we share it with every other biological organism.

So the real deleterious effects to our health come from the Type 2 stressors?

Precisely.

Can you explain those?

A Type 2 stressor is the more familiar one to us. Very few things in our environment are genuine threats to our physical well-being. However, there exist a tremendous number of internal and external emotional demands that are not immediate, identifiable, or resolvable in the short run and which affect us daily. For example, it could be something as simple as a source of noise we're not even consciously aware of, though it is creating a state of arousal in us. Other concerns might be interpersonal difficulties with people, pressure at work, time pressures and deadlines, family problems, or economic difficulties. All these concerns translate into almost the exact same physiological response from the body as would a more imminent threat. In other words, our body tends to respond to stress naively. It can't tell the difference between a real physical threat, such as a car coming at us, or something we only perceive to be such a threat... such as losing our job. These two events create a virtually identical biochemical response in the body. The problem is that, because the difficulty is a cumulative response to Type 2 stressors. The period of arousal becomes protracted, and eventually this protracted stress response becomes a symptom of disease.

Can you cite some examples?

A perfectly normal response to stress is for your heart rate to increase. That's fine for a short period of time. But if it becomes protracted, the result might be tachycardia. If that situation persists and the tachycardia remains undiagnosed, the heart might become further compromised. Another common reaction to stress is for the muscles to clench. The skeletal system becomes rigid. That's fine for combat, since you wouldn't be so easy to push over by the adversary. But if that clenching isn't released, you will begin to develop musculoskeletal pain, compression in the lower back, spasms, ticks, and tension headaches. It is this protracted and chronic stress reaction that is literally the killer.

Now we also go through a period of compensatory rebound from this kind of consistent stress. We call these rebounds by a lot of names or conditions. They can manifest as headaches, depression, or even full-blown heart attacks. In other words, the rebound could be an extreme physical disorder requiring hospitalization. The point I'm making is that the body can't continue with this sort of protracted response. Biologically, we will ultimately break at some weak link... and we all have at least one if not more such weak links.

Would prolonged stress also negatively affect the functioning of the immune system?

Absolutely. One of the things that results from chronic stress is that the immune system becomes depressed. The immune system is critical to our health, since it performs two vital functions within the body. For one thing it serves as a surveillance system, guarding the body against either bacteria or viruses. Secondly, there is a theory—and it is *only* a theory, though it's being increasingly accepted—called immunological surveillance. This theory posits that the immune system also maintains internal surveillance systems regulating aberrant or abnormal cell division. So if the body's cells begin to divide abnormally beyond a certain point, the immune system will attack those cells and rid the body of them so they can't progress into a malignancy. During periods of stress, some of the stress hormones—such as corticosteroids and espinephrine—depress the

46   activity of the immune system. This makes a person more susceptible to infection or to the development of cancer. There's also research coming to light now that stress may be a contributing factor which diminishes the immune system's capacity to fight off the HIV virus— the AIDS virus.

Do personality factors interact with stress factors? Do certain personality types react more poorly to prolonged stress?

That's a good question, and unfortunately, it's one that's difficult to answer. Probably the most obvious contributing personality type to disease that's reasonably well-documented is the Type A personality, who is predisposed to heart disease. The Type A person is time-driven, aggressive, and angry inside. He harbors repressed anger bordering on rage.

Now the most important thing to remember is that this Type A behavior is only one of a number of factors that predispose a person to heart disease. You also have to take into consideration a person's genetic history, dietary cholesterol, serum cholesterol level, and so on. The idea that a particular personality style predisposes a person to a specific disease is emphatically wrong... such as that a person who's rigid is going to get arthritis, or that a person who is hot-tempered is going to get heart disease, or that a depressed and inwardly dwelling person is prone to get cancer. Although these are influences, the mind/body system is certainly more complex than that.

We've been talking about how the mind can make a person sick, but now I'd like to discuss whether the mind can cure. What are the best procedures a person can use to overcome the effects of personal stress?

That's an important issue. In fact, how the positive states of mind and emotions can create beneficial effects—both physically and mentally—is of greater interest to me than disease. We know so little about the possibilities. We now have a reasonable accumulation of information about mind/body interactions and how they can create illness, yet we know almost nothing about how these same factors can create states of health. The critical matter is: What would be an ideal response to stress?

What is your response to that question?

I think it involves a four-stage process, which is based on classic learning theory. It's the same as learning how we do everything, from tying our shoes to higher order differential equations. In essence, what we need to do is identify the stresses in our lives clearly and honestly. We have to identify our *specific* stressors. So the first stage in the process is a simple act of identification. The second stage is to take a physical break from our usual chronic and negative response to that stressor. For example, say that you chronically feel yourself in a competitive situation with a colleague at work. Instead of arguing with that person, take a physical break from the conflict. These breaks represent various forms of relaxation. So it could be a period of meditation, ranging from Zen to transcendental meditation, or it could be doing some yoga. It could also be biofeedback or simply Zazen breathing. Other procedures might include the practice of progressive muscular relaxation or autogenic training. Anything that works for you is satisfactory.

Now for the third stage. Once you have learned to become physically quiet, this creates a potential for mental quiet. We're no longer reflexively responding to the person, or the situation, or the negative emotion that is causing us problems. And one of the most powerful tools we can use at this point is to engage in specific ways of quieting the mind... by entering the higher consciousness dimensions of meditation, which could be by the use of a mantra—or any other word. It doesn't have to be in Sanskrit! It could also be a prayer, a poem, or simply contemplating the name of a person, a sound, or an image. In their more complex stage, these practices will evolve into the practice of visual imagery. During this state we can begin to rehearse alternative responses to the stress.

Which means that a person can rehearse these strategies and practice them at home in order to anticipate the stressor when it occurs?

Precisely. While in this stage of mental quiet, you're not anxious and are freed from your usual automatic responses. That's where the process of visualization becomes very powerful, allowing you to see and to rehearse alternatives to the situation that has you in difficulty.

And the fourth stage?

The fourth stage is what can be called empowerment, which is where the individual takes a new action. For example, if fighting traffic while driving to work is bothering you, you leave fifteen minutes

48 earlier rather than always being on the freeway fighting for your life. Or when your office colleague comes in and makes his usual antagonistic, snide remark, you don't respond the way you usually do. The chain of stress has now been broken. In other words, what was stressful last week isn't *this* week. So you've changed your orientation, you've changed your worldview, and you've changed responses. You've actually changed your consciousness to a great degree. People can change their lives in a much more positive direction by employing this essentially very simple four-stage learning process.

You've been emphasizing stresses that typically occur in the workplace. I understand that your recent concern has been directed toward the health hazards—both psychological and physical—that exist there. Could you elaborate on your work in this area?

Beginning about six or seven years ago, people who were very successful began coming to me as patients. These were people who had successful careers but who were feeling unfulfilled or stressed at work. They would make comments such as, "No matter how much I like what I'm doing, there's a tremendous strain involved with it." So initially, I began to work with individuals and then with departments—specifically at the credit card division of a major bank—to develop stress management programs. That work has evolved over time and led me to write my most recent book, *Healthy People in Unhealthy Places.* Now that title really sums up how a lot of people feel. There are people who might be eating right, meditating and running, and maintaining a good family life. But then they go to work! I don't know anyone who simply works an eight-hour day anymore. People are working ten hours a day now, sometimes, five, six, or even seven days a week. What that means is that work-related stress is potentially the greatest health hazard we are facing today.

Other than conflicts with coworkers, what kinds of physical and psychological stressors are today's employees facing?

If you look at the physical environment of many offices and workplaces, there's diminished privacy. There's also poor lighting, there can be toxic emissions from the way some of the buildings are constructed, or there can be inadequate recycling of the air. That's especially true of today's highly sealed, energy-efficient buildings. We could add to this list the use of video display terminals, where people work for long periods of time in sedentary positions. These all constitute a set of potential—and I want to keep emphasizing potential — hazards to the mind and body.

Now to me, the interesting thing is that some of our major corporations—AT&T, Johnson & Johnson, Tenneco, Xerox, and IBM—began to develop what they call "health promotion" programs about three or four years ago. These were simply programs whereby their employees could learn skills—such as the one I just described for managing stress—to help remain healthy, productive, and in high-performance condition. That's all very exciting because you're working with an essentially highly motivated, educated, and relatively healthy population... a population that wants to get even better.

I take it that both the employer and the worker benefit from the program.

The corporation wins because it has healthy employees, while the employees win because they feel better and less strained. Very often there are rewards—such as forms of financial incentive—built right into the program. So there's an incentive for the employee to stay healthy.

So you feel the corporations can gain financially from instituting these kinds of programs?

The evidence is getting better in this respect, although it wasn't very good until recently. These programs don't show cost effectiveness in less than three years, but they have now finally been around long enough and are beginning to show cost benefits at AT&T, Tenneco, Johnson & Johnson, and Blue Cross. Our corporations are learning to benefit by reducing the psychological and physical risk factors in the workplace. When you reduce smoking, reduce stress, improve diet, introduce exercise, conduct early screening for high blood pressure, use mammography or progressive cancer screening— when you reduce risk factors through the voluntary efforts of your employees, you start to see less disease. As you see less disease you start paying fewer medical bills, since most corporations pay for their own medical costs.

Let me interject one thing, though. These programs were not originally initiated by these companies in order to save money. They were

50   initiated by companies who genuinely cared about their employees. Rather cynically, some people like to look back and say that these companies were just trying to squeeze more from the workers. But that wasn't their original purpose. They were genuinely interested because somebody, usually a chief executive, had a personal experience with improving his or her health and decided to make that benefit available in the company.

I also understand that you are involved in a lengthy study to develop holistic health programs for the work environment.

Right now [1987] we are in the second year of a five-year program at the University of California School of Medicine, San Francisco. When I say "we," I'm referring to a number of our faculty members in the Division of Internal Medicine at the school. The purpose of the program is to develop and *evaluate*—that "evaluate" is important to emphasize—the efficacy of health promotion programs from both health and financial viewpoints.

It involved fifteen major corporations which, with a single exception, are all located in northern California. The reason for that is that we're a real working group. We meet together quarterly to identify areas of mutual interest. To give you an example: Bank of America was engaged in a large blood pressure screening program for its employees. We, on the other hand, had expertise regarding what to do with those people with high blood pressure once they were identified, to lessen their chances of disease. So we collaborated, wrote a grant proposal, and now we're conducting a joint program in the behavioral management of hypertension with a three-year grant from the National Institutes of Health. And that's just one example.

What other companies are involved, and how would they benefit from such a program?

The companies that are now involved include Bank of America, Apple, Levi-Strauss, Hewlett-Packard, Chevron, Safeway, Lockheed, AT&T, and Shackley Corporation, among others. These are, of course, well-known companies. We begin by identifying a problem area in the workplace, and then we work with the company to develop a program to deal with it. Once this program has been developed, the other companies can either adopt the same program for their environment, work with the other company to share the program, or simply decide to forget it. These programs might range from the stress management program we've developed for Levi-Strauss, to a mammography screening program for breast cancer we're developing with Apple, to the hypertension program with Bank of America. We meet four times a year at one of the corporate sites, and the companies get to see what these programs are all about.

Has the program been successful?

It has been very successful. Health care in the near future, five or ten years from now, is going to be increasingly governed by the kinds of programs that corporations decide to provide for their employees. Corporations right now control 40–43 percent of the total medical budget in the United States. That means 40–43 percent of $450 billion a year. These companies are beginning to become much more active in moving toward disease prevention while still providing appropriate and high quality medical care for their employees.

Are there any other benefits from these kinds of programs?

The fact is that the employees derive a great deal of satisfaction beyond the basic health benefits of a particular program. For example, we had a stress management program at one company while it was undergoing a merger, and the program helped. But just knowing something was available to the employees during this period of time apparently benefited even those workers who chose not to enroll. There's an intangible benefit that is becoming increasingly important.

What do you see for the future of holistic health care in the workplace?

It is growing and expanding, and for a number of reasons. Because of government legislation and some very complex changes in the way medical expenses are reimbursed, this 40–43 percent portion of the total United States medical budget is going to grow. Estimates are that as much as seventy percent of our medical care will be absorbed by the workplace by the year 2000. A second factor to remember is that our entire population is aging, and all chronic disease is age-related. The older we get, the more chronic disease manifests. If we can't manage the amount of chronic disease we have right now, think of the future. Already there are major insurance carriers that are bankrupt. Hospitals are going out of business because they can't

52   manage the amount of chronic disease we have in our young population at the present time. So our corporations will have to take a more
active role in preventing a substantial proportion of what we see as
disease.

**I'd like to finish by leaving the world of business and discuss
the purely metaphysical implications of your work. Do you
think that engaging in spiritual exercises or entering onto the
"spiritual path" can itself be a beneficial, stress-reducing
activity... whether for an employee, an executive, or a labor-
er?**

That's an excellent question. There is very good evidence that a
strong sense of purpose in life helps a person. That sense of purpose
may not be what someone identifies as a particular religion or religious belief. But when a person has the sense of a purposive, evolving universe in which he or she has an active purposive role, the
resulting sense of empowerment can positively influence his life. It
isn't only a powerful mitigator against disease, but there is some indication that it can enhance the immune system as well.

Let me give you an example. One researcher at Harvard University
has discovered what is called the "Mother Teresa" effect. He showed
some students a rather violent, warlike film and found afterward that
their immune systems were depressed. Then he showed them a docu-
mentary of Mother Teresa ministering to the children of Calcutta, and
the students' immune systems were apparently enhanced by viewing
it. That's the Mother Teresa effect. So there are actually conditions
under which we can enhance our immunological response, and these
conditions evolve from faith, hope, optimism, love, altruism, and
compassion. In fact, what we may very well see in the future is a
whole science of the effects of the positive emotions on our lives.
That's very likely and it will certainly be most interesting to see what
happens.

2 | RIGHT LIVING AS THERAPY

AN INTERVIEW WITH
LEWIS M. ANDREWS, PH.D.

B   I   O   G   R   A   P   H   Y

Lewis M. Andrews, Ph.D., was born in New York and educated at Princeton University and Stanford University. He earned his doctorate in psychology at the Union Graduate School in Cincinnati, Ohio. He has conducted seminars and workshops on ethical therapy at Villanova University, the University of Hartford, Duke University, and many hospitals around the country. A recent research fellow at the Yale University Divinity School, he is currently a visiting scholar at Columbia University. He is the coauthor of a textbook on psychology and a trade book on biofeedback, and his most recent book is *To Thine Own Self Be True*, which deals with the relationship between ethical values and emotional health.

I probably never would have heard of Dr. Lewis M. Andrews but for the ever alert eye of John Neindorf, the former editor of *Science of Mind* magazine. He had found a new book called *To Thine Own Self Be True* by Dr. Andrews, which suggested that teaching moral values should be part of psychotherapy. Such a suggestion is anathema to the way much therapy, especially psychoanalytically based, is undertaken in the United States. He even proffered that psychotherapy *without* such implicit values could be detrimental. The iconoclastic premise of the book immediately roused my curiosity so I read it during a plane trip to Atlanta the following week.

Dr. Andrews lives on the East Coast, but as luck (synchronicity?) would have it, he was due in Los Angeles in a few weeks to promote the book and was scheduled for a radio interview within a few miles of my home. I met Dr. Andrews at the station. It turned out that we had several colleagues in common and the short drive to my house gave us a few moments to get acquainted. We spent half the time conducting the interview, while Dr. Andrews—a bibliophile—spent the rest examining my library.

D. SCOTT ROGO: What do you mean when you say in your book *To Thine Own Self Be True* that psychology can be the cause—as much as the cure—of our emotional problems?

LEWIS M. ANDREWS: I mean there is a growing body of evidence which suggests that conventional psychotherapy isn't all it's represented to be. For example, there was a study conducted at the Kaiser hospitals about ten years ago. They had one hundred patients who were asking to go into therapy, but only about fifty therapists were available. So they divided the potential patients into two groups. The group that went into psychotherapy didn't do any better in the long run than the people on the waiting list! A number of other studies carried out over the years have shown similar results. There is even some statistical evidence that people going into therapy do worse than if they had not gone into therapy.

That's quite an indictment, but it obviously doesn't apply to all therapy—particularly the kind you advocate.

That's exactly right. It is an indictment of some traditional forms of psychotherapy, such as behaviorism, psychoanalysis, and psychoanalytically derived psychotherapy, which are considered value-free.

And what is value-free therapy?

The easiest way to define it is to look at its history, particularly against a background of the 1920s, when psychologists—the Ph.D.s within the university system—and the psychiatrists—who organized psychoanalysis in this country—became organized. That's when the profession first came into being and when licensure was issued. That's also when the American Medical Association decided they were going to take over psychoanalysis and make it a medical discipline. So they developed a curriculum and got the State of New York to decree that nobody could be a psychoanalyst without an M.D. degree. The psychologists did something similar at the university level by setting up programs in clinical psychology.

While this was being accomplished, both the psychologists and the psychiatrists were very suspicious of religion. Organized religion, of course, has been the traditional repository of ethical and moral values over the centuries, but these pioneers in the field also felt that religion was the cause of many people's emotional problems. Sigmund Freud, for instance, believed most mental illness was a function of repression, and psychiatrists and psychologists associated repression with conservative religious thinking. So they decided their field was going to have nothing to do with anything religious or anything that even sounded religious or spiritual. The field prided itself on being value-free.

Something else that contributed to the problem was that this was the time of the Scopes "monkey" trial, where a teacher in Tennessee who was presenting Darwin's theory of evolution had been put on trial, principally because his teachings were so deeply in conflict with the prevailing conservative religious views. This only increased the prejudice among certain educated people against religion.

56 **Why do you object to the value-free approach to helping people with their problems?**

Because it doesn't seem to work. As I show in *To Thine Own Self Be True*, the only thing that really seems related to people getting well in therapy is their returning to basic ethical and spiritual values. As the Swiss psychiatrist C. G. Jung said, and I'm paraphrasing here, nobody ever really gets well who doesn't go back to the basics of spiritual values. These are the values that lie at the heart of all the world's great religions and philosophies. In fact, when I began researching my book, it had a different title. It was to be called *The Eternal Therapy*, and my goal was to identify the common psychotherapy at the heart of all the great religions and philosophies.

Now when you look at these religions, you find that, in terms of prescribing a psychological regimen for health, they share a number of similarities. The three similarities that seem to be universal are greater honesty, greater tolerance of other people, and the belief in something greater than the self. If a person were religious he'd call that "something" God, while a person more scientifically oriented and without spiritual inclinations would call it, perhaps, "trusting your intuition." But it is still the belief in some sort of inner power greater than yourself.

Interestingly, to believe in "something greater" is the same prescription the really good therapists come to respect. As I said, that's what Jung regarded as necessary for mental health and even what Sigmund Freud said—even though his writings about it have been greatly distorted over the years.

What do you believe makes a really good therapist?

A number of studies on the effectiveness of psychotherapy have indicated that the only factor that really seems to correlate with a patient's getting well is the character of the therapist. It's not the therapist's training, it's not where he went to school, or whether he's Freudian or a behaviorist, but whether he has good values himself—and can convey those values to his patients. That's the kind of therapist who is most likely to have a positive effect on his or her patient's life.

Since ethical therapy is based on religious and spiritual values, how does it differ from old-fashioned pastoral counseling?

In some respects there's not a lot of difference. But in pastoral counseling there's frequently somebody coming out of a particular denomination. So the counseling, while it usually deals with these same basic values, tends to be oriented around a particular religion. But when we're talking about ethical therapy, we're really talking about the highest common factor of all religions and philosophies. So we're not denominational in ethical therapy, not concerned with the differences that could distinguish a Jew from a Christian or Buddhist, or a Presbyterian from a Congregationalist or Methodist. We're looking at what is universal, but we're also looking at what is scientific and testable. There's now a growing body of scientific research which indicates that learning these values makes the difference in a patient's trying to overcome problems.

So I take it that you feel a psychologist should personally have a strong spiritual sense and commitment.

To be effective, yes. Alan Bergin of Brigham Young University has reported a fascinating study in which he surveyed 425 practicing psychologists, psychiatrists, and social workers. He asked them what they did in the privacy of their offices that got people well. He found that the vast majority of them, in spite of their conventional education, came to value very highly the things I've talked about—that is, the importance of people becoming more honest, more tolerant, and coming to believe in something greater than themselves, hopefully something spiritual. The most fascinating aspect of Bergin's study in my opinion is that a high percentage of practicing therapists in this country are members of an organized church and are actively involved in it. That's something you wouldn't know from reading anything about psychology.

What specific change in life, or the way we go about the business of living, can most people adopt to live a more fulfilling and less stressful existence?

If I were going to summarize it, I would say that the place to start is with the problem of manipulation. That's what we're most aware of, because I think we all have manipulative tendencies. For example, we think we can get somebody to do what we want by flattering them. Or we feel we can advance our own personal circumstance by withholding information from somebody else. Or we tend to put on our

58 "best face" in certain situations even though that entails some sort of minor deception.

We should start taking the risk of being a little more honest in those situations where we're tempted to manipulate other people or to tell a little white lie. This doesn't mean revealing the intimate details of your personal life for everyone to inspect, or even being open about everything. I think that's too much to ask in the beginning. But we should experiment with being a little more honest in our day-to-day interactions in order to see the result it has. What we begin to discover is that it has a very positive result and good things begin to happen, though not in the ways we'd predict. The more we act in this way, the more we become capable of being honest. We learn that it has value and a positive impact in our lives... a type of impact we were never previously aware of.

Another important thing is learning to restrain our hostile thoughts and judgments, particularly the judgments. Remember that wonderful story about Ben Franklin?

The one about humility?

Yes. You'll recall that Franklin went to a church and heard a sermon on morals. He was so put off by the dryness of it that he decided to look at it from a more scientific point of view. So he made a list of all the virtues he could come up with—charity, forgiveness, honesty, chastity, and so forth. He decided to devote a week to practicing each of these virtues to see what effect they would have on his life.

He was in the middle of preparing this little experiment when he was talking to a Quaker friend of his who said something like, "Ben, there's one virtue that's not on your list. It's the one you really need to work on. It's humility." Franklin was a very proud man, even arrogant—especially in his way of speaking. So he put humility on his list and that became the key which really turned his life around. He admits this in his autobiography. He was never able to get over his arrogant thinking, because he always felt he was superior to other people, but he was able to get over his habitual use of such words as *indubitably, undoubtedly,* or *surely*—the kinds of words we often use when we're speaking in an arrogant way or when we're being critical of somebody else.

Is there anything else you would suggest?

As I mentioned before, I think it is important to give increasing validity to our intuitive feelings. Every day we come up against situations where we're faced with choices. The choice that is logical represents one of our options, but something inside of us often says we should make a different choice.

When we get older, we begin to realize that this intuitive voice is usually right. So, when and if we find ourselves in situations where we're torn between what seems to be the logical way to respond and what we intuitively feel, let's give ourselves a pause and come down on the side of intuition a little more frequently. I think that has an enormous healing effect on people's lives.

Could you cite an example from your own experience of how being less judgmental actually helped somebody with a problem?

There is the interesting instance of a boy who was very rebellious and judgmental toward his father. He was depressed and he came into therapy because he was having all kinds of problems. He was a cutup in school. He liked to think he was a real rebel. But it was pointed out to him that his rebelliousness was really no rebellion at all. Even though he seemed to be rebelling, his behavior was completely predictable. If his father wanted him to get an A in history, for example, the kid would fail the class. But if his father didn't care whether his son did well in, say, art history, the boy would get an A. You could know exactly what the boy was going to do by looking at what his father wanted. The point was made that he needed to stop judging his father, which he did, and that really turned his life around.

Is ethical therapy being actually used anywhere? Is there evidence as to its effectiveness?

That's a really good question, because when I discuss ethical therapy, people generally ask, "Where is this practiced?" And I suggest that they look at programs such as Alcoholics Anonymous, where they'll find almost the purest expression of what I'm referring to. Alcoholics Anonymous is, in fact, a nondenominational spiritual therapy which places emphasis on honesty, tolerance, intuitive self-reliance, and some sort of higher power. It is certainly the most effective treatment for alcoholism.

What's so fascinating about AA is that its model is beginning to be

60   expanded, so you now have Cocaine Anonymous, Overeaters Anonymous, Sexaholics Anonymous, and so on. If you were to add all the people in AA — which is an estimated two million—to all the people in other, related programs, you'd have more clients in these programs than in all the therapists' offices combined. It is the single most successful therapeutic approach in the country, but you would not find it mentioned in a single psychiatric textbook.

What evidence can you cite that the attitudes which result from living an ethically ordered life are psychologically and physically beneficial?

In regard to attitudes themselves, the most dramatic work I know of is that of Carl Thoresen of Stanford University with recovering heart attack patients. In his studies of people who have suffered heart attacks, he found that they tend to be hostile and resentful people, and he divided them into two groups. The people in one group were given the traditional therapy for coronary patients, such as to cut down on cholesterol, get more exercise, and so forth. The people in the other group were also given these instructions but, in addition, they were told that their attitudes were killing them. They were given a series of little phrases to use whenever a difficult situation came up, such as "Let it go" or "Let it pass" or "Nothing's worth getting upset about." The people in this latter group had a significantly lower incidence of second heart attacks.

And in my book I talk a lot about the negative effects of hostility, resentment, and judgmental attitudes. I point out that these attitudes not only lead to depression but to a literal collapse of the body. We know from research carried out ten years ago, for example, that people who are extremely hostile and judgmental tend to suffer from coronaries more frequently than less hostile, less resentful people. Being able to get a grip on our judgmental and hostile attitudes is so powerful that it heals us emotionally and it has a large impact on our physical health.

You write in your book that a strong sense of ethics has a powerful relationship to success in business, and I thought that was very provocative. Can you explain what you mean?

It is provocative because we tend to think about business only in terms of Wall Street scandals, and it's certainly true that there are people in business who are unethical. But it's also true that there are unethical people in every field. There are unethical therapists, unethical teachers, and so on.

But if you look for what makes for success and what executives value in their workers, ethics is very high on the list. *The Wall Street Journal* did a study of executives in terms of their hiring practices. What is it they look for when promoting people? The executives placed honesty and character at the top of the list. There is a reason for this, especially in big business and corporations, because these people manage enormous sums of money and have great responsibility to their stockholders, pension-fund holders, and so forth. The men and women who run these companies don't get trusted unless they are people of very high character.

I think that's true in all areas of life. I think cream rises to the top, so to speak, and the people who get to the top in any field are people who, for the most part, inspire the trust and confidence of their coworkers.

Why do you feel that teaching such commonsense values has become so controversial in psychology?

There are probably a couple of reasons. The first, as I mentioned earlier, involves where psychology is coming from. The field has equated the issue of values with dogmatic religion and therefore automatically assumes that working with values is unscientific. That's not true, of course, since you can easily test the scientific benefits of strong personal values. In *To Thine Own Self Be True*, I recount many experiments which show a positive relationship between people's values and their emotional health. But there's been a prejudice within psychology against such an approach.

The other reason is, in my opinion, that psychologists have a vested economic interest in ignoring the relationship between values and emotional health. That is a startling thing to say, but recently I've come to understand it more clearly. I have recognized that as traditional psychologists become more involved with discussing spiritual values, they begin more and more to acknowledge that therapy is a spiritual enterprise. Psychologists, however, are enormously dependent upon what's called third-party reimbursement from both the

62   state and federal governments. Now, you really don't need to go to school or get a license to practice therapy. Anyone can do it. But you do need a license to get the third-party reimbursement, the part of a patient's bill paid by the state or federal government or by the insurance companies.

So, if therapists begin to acknowledge that they are, in effect, teaching spiritual values, they come close to violating the First Amendment in regard to separation of church and state. The issue is something like this: If engaging in psychotherapy is a spiritual enterprise, can the state legitimately subsidize it without being involved in subsidizing religion? So I believe we're dealing here with the unconscious awareness—and I stress the word *unconscious*—of psychologists that if they talk about what really works in therapy, they'll have to deal with the possibility of a massive economic reorganization. And I don't think they are prepared for that.

What advice would you give to people who aren't in therapy, who feel essentially healthy and live basically ethical lives, but who are bored with everything?

That's an interesting question, because it's based on what a person means by "ethical," and even more generally it involves what people mean by any of the high-sounding words they use. For instance, lots of people talk about ethics and think they're very ethical, but in fact are extremely judgmental and intolerant. Often the people who claim to be ethical are the ones who are the least ethical. Their ethical concerns can be masks for their own intolerance. You see the same thing in relationships where honesty is really used to hurt someone. You say something you know is going to hurt another person and claim you are just being honest. Well, you aren't just being honest; you're actually going in for the kill.

So when people tell me they're leading an ethical life and are bored, I suggest that they take a closer look at their values. People who lead an ethical life—which to me means a spiritual life—don't get bored, because spirituality is intrinsically creative and satisfying in its own right.

3 | MUSIC AND YOUR HEALTH

AN INTERVIEW WITH STEVEN HALPERN

B   I   O   G   R   A   P   H   Y

Steven Halpern is generally considered to be this country's foremost pioneer in the development and promotion of New Age music. He has devoted his life to the study of the healthful and uplifting power and sound of music, and has received international recognition for his contributions. His lifelong interest in music became focused when he began formal training, at the age of nine. His studies continued and expanded through college, where he earned his tuition as a performing musician and where his interest in alternative musical forms began to develop. He is the composer, producer, and principal recording artist of over forty-five albums, tapes, and compact discs, including his famous "Anti-Frantic Alternative" tm series of recordings for relaxation and for listening pleasure. He is also the coauthor (with Louis Savary) of *Sound Health: Music and Sounds That Make Us Whole.*

M usic has always served an important role in my life, but I never thought that my musical training and education in music would contribute to my psychological interests. For many years, I worked in both parapsychology and in Los Angeles's busy music industry, with relatively few of my peers in each realm knowing of my other occupation! But the 1970s brought with them a new understanding of both the neurology and therapeutic value of music. Music therapy even evolved as a legitimate field within psychology.

Steven Halpern has been an eminent spokesman for the healing power of music, and conversely, he has warned of the serious effects of noise pollution. This interview became a double pleasure when I learned that he and I share a similar problem. Being sensitive to sounds and noises, both of us are victims of noise pollution—we simply cannot stand environmental noises. Much of our meeting, which was scheduled to explore his role as a composer of "healing music," focused on the quietest refrigerator on the market, the car with the softest engine noise, and other mutual concerns. It was an ironic meeting, however, since the scene was probably the noisiest place in modern society. I caught Steven en route to San Diego, so the interview was taped in a lounge at Los Angeles International Airport.

D. SCOTT ROGO: Many people know you only through your recordings and may not be aware that you believe there is more to what you call "sound health" than just listening to relaxing music.

STEVEN HALPERN: That's right. Composing and recording uplifting music has certainly been a major focus of my work, but I've always been involved in a larger spectrum of sound-related issues. For example, I am very much concerned with environmental noise pollution.

When I travel around the country lecturing, I find increasing numbers of people who are also aware of the problem. Let me give you an example. In my workshops, one of the first things I do is to ask people to take a sound inventory—for example, by just listening to the sounds going on in their homes. Typically, the first sound most people hear is the refrigerator. But they've never really *listened* to it before, never really felt it in their bodies. While that's only a single example, it is a noise that usually permeates the entire house and interferes with meaningful relaxation—often while people are sleeping or trying to meditate. It's like sitting on an acoustic thumbtack.

Could you cite another example?

There are hundreds. Yesterday for two solid hours, there were gardeners in my neighborhood using power mowers and leaf blowers that made the whole house shake! I couldn't talk on the phone, my brain stopped functioning, and my irritation levels rose dramatically. As I point out in my book *Sound Health*, one of the problems with there being so few laws on the books concerning noise pollution is that the sound level has increased significantly year by year. The fire spotters in Mozart's day could shout from the roofs of buildings and be heard, but nowadays even sirens have to be louder and louder to be effective.

So the problem is definitely getting worse?

Yes, international studies have shown that the noise level in the environment is rising a decibel a year. The human body has just not been designed to deal with such continuous loud noise. More and more we are being assaulted by these sounds—by jet planes flying overhead, the neighbor's TV and stereo, the construction going on down the block, and so forth. Even if they aren't explosively loud, they are still taking a toll on our hearing. When I'm in New York, for example, my friends shout at me even when I'm sitting three feet from them. They've had to acclimate themselves to the environmental din of the city and don't realize their own obvious hearing loss. Having known the same people for ten years, I recognize this change as an immediate piece of evidence that something is wrong.

This problem is especially evident in restaurants, where the music is often so loud and fast that it makes digestion and conversation impossible. The volume in movie theaters is also getting louder and louder.

66 **Do you feel this situation can be changed?**

I do, and that's one of the reasons I'm involved in this work. My goal is to raise people's awareness that this problem is developing, so we can have a chance to do something about it. Some experts are predicting universal deafness if this trend continues. Part of what we can do is to encourage political action, so we can get laws on the books limiting the noise pollution created by certain trucks, jets, and construction sites. And that's what is actually beginning to happen. As sound awareness is being raised, people are beginning to take charge of the environment, saying enough is enough. The quality of our lives is more important than another truck on the streets or the noisy construction of another building.

You referred to noise pollution in the home as well as in the outside environment. Do you feel the noise level inside the home can actually be dangerous?

There certainly is a cumulative effect from the sounds of refrigerators, dishwashers, vacuum cleaners, and so on. It can be dangerous in the following respect: If we wish to be healthy, happy, and efficient working people, anything that interferes with our natural state of wellness will have a deleterious effect on us. Sound pollution gets on our nerves, whether it's loud sounds such as jet planes or the subtle sounds of air conditioners or refrigerators. They keep people more tense than they need to be. And to deal with that tension, people tend to reach for drugs—legal or illegal—or tune it out with television. So even if the sounds are not destructive in terms of their decibel levels, they are certainly nonhealthful.

We know that relaxation is a prerequisite for letting the body heal. So if your body never gets a chance to relax, it is always going to be off-key. The ramifications for our psychological, physical, and spiritual health are obvious.

Do you feel this danger comes from some forms of music as well as from environmental noises?

That's a good question. Much of the music that is popular today has not been designed with the health of the listener in mind. In fact, I think that's a clear understatement. The rhythmic structure of a lot of this music is opposed to the natural rhythm of the heart. That in itself stresses the heart and weakens the body.

One of the people who has done pioneering research on this problem is Dr. John Diamond. As a medical professional, he has conducted a lot of research with behavioral kinestheology and pinpointed the fact that these rhythms have a stressful effect on the body. The other obvious problem with today's music is the volume at which people listen to it. However, even if you listen to loud classical music, you are going to have a problem. The sound levels available today at concerts, through home stereo systems, and even through portable walk-around tape recorders can get up to 120 decibels. The human ear is simply not designed to handle that kind of volume and it can cause irreversible, cumulative damage that results in a self-perpetuating cycle. As you lose your hearing, you start raising the volume to get the same feeling you got before. Of course, the more you raise the volume, the more damage you do.

As I travel around the country, I meet many audiologists who report that their clientele have changed radically over the last fifteen years—from mostly people over fifty-five to people who, in fifty percent of the cases, are under thirty. These people are clearly the victims of this type of self-abuse. And those numbers are misleading, since they represent only the people who are willing to admit to having a problem.

In your book you state, "a regular diet of certain kinds of music and sound can help our bodies and minds to achieve higher levels of health." Can you explain what you mean?

In terms of what I call "sound nutrition," I think we should select our musical diet somewhat like we select our food. We ought not to select only one kind of music, but should partake of a varied diet. Within that diet, my prescription suggests that some music should be used to let the body relax. In those states, the body is able to tune and heal itself. That's important because, say medical researchers, the body is a programmed and self-rectifying organism that needs a change to get back into attunement with itself. Just giving yourself something like five minutes a day of some form of psychotechnology to let the body heal is going to be beneficial. There are many ways of getting back to this state, and one of the simplest is listening to beautiful music.

But simply listening to relaxing music is not the goal of sound nutrition, nor is its goal to listen exclusively to strongly emotional or cathartic music. That's why I suggest a varied diet. No one genre can supply everything you need.

68 Just how does a person choose the most specifically healthful music?

That's a tough question, since everyone is unique and individual. But certain generalizations can be made. By virtue of being human organisms living on this planet, we have certain vibrations in common. Harmonics of eight cycles per second, for instance, tend to entrain—to bring about—very positive biologically and genetically preprogrammed responses in the body. There are ways of stimulating alpha waves — those brain waves that occur when a person is relaxed—by playing music that resonates with such harmonics. These harmonics may be engineered right into compositions—such as in my *Spectrum Suite* or *Crystal Suite*—which trigger the production of alpha waves. By providing the proper rhythmic context, such music will help the body to properly balance itself. You can test this situation by getting your brain waves checked with biofeedback equipment or by testing muscle tension.

Is there a less complicated way of telling?

There's something I call the full-belly effect. I sometimes test a particular composition after I've eaten a big meal. If it interferes with my digestion it doesn't qualify as relaxational. Music that may not be good for you can give you a pain in the back or neck. Or it might begin hurting your stomach or cause your breath to become shallow, rapid, or irregular. For example, much rap and dance music uses artificial drum machines that create stutter rhythms that are arhythmic—rhythms that you never hear outside a cardiac arrest ward in a hospital! Such music can certainly cause irregularities in the listener's heart rhythms. We have to balance such music by listening to some sort of healing music. So the ultimate test is to be attentive to your own body. If your body feels good and your breathing becomes more regular when you listen to certain music, then the music is probably in keeping with the natural needs of the body.

Now there might be a time on Saturday night when you want to dance and boogie, a time when otherwise unhealthful music might be appropriate. But in general, listening to that kind of music while doing anything else is like pushing the gas and brake pedals of your car simultaneously.

What do you feel are some of the most positive benefits of listening to music?

We're finding through research that, at its core, listening to beautiful music tends to release endorphins—chemicals in the brain that cause a sense of well-being and relief from pain. As the research continues to be published, we find that this is one of the wonderful ways the body maintains higher levels of functioning. We all know that listening to beautiful music feels good. This isn't anything you have to intellectualize. You can tell as a result of your direct experience. In fact, while listening to certain music, you can break down the barriers and get beyond the structure into the pure sound, so you *become* the music. The music can help bring you back in touch with your own Higher Nature, to the Creator. A lot of great classical music was designed for just that purpose.

In regard to the field of New Age music, we recognize that it is music specifically created to help people tune in to their Higher Nature. You see, the body is not impressed by complexity. You don't necessarily have to be knocked out by the music, but the music—sometimes through its subtleties—carries you into a state where your body can be more effectively played by the Cosmos.

Do you believe music can also be used as a specific treatment for stress?

Certainly. Music is legal, nonaddictive, and you can use it in the home. There's no question about it now, and that's partly what got me into the field in the first place some fifteen years ago. I was a good, solid Type A person coming from New York and I was already exhibiting some of the telltale symptoms of stress. I was looking for something that would combine my background in music with my backgrounds in psychology and sociology and which I could use myself. That way I wouldn't have to go to somebody else's office every time I got stressed out. In answer to prayer and meditation, I started hearing and knowing about the music I'm playing now.

Since that time I've been able to get my music into many hospitals. What they find is that, independent of all sorts of demographics and psychographics, music such as my "Anti-Frantic Alternative"[tm] relaxes people. The music accomplishes this goal in several ways. It doesn't have the pounding beat of most music. That fact in itself lets

70   the body settle down. Secondly, it doesn't have some of the structural imperatives that most compositions have which rivet your attention and focus your energy on the music rather than on yourself.

Studies have been conducted for the last fifty years showing that certain music helps people relax. But now we have more sophisticated techniques for measuring relaxation, such as biofeedback and brain wave recordings. We now know the specific physiological parameters of relaxation and we know that the right music can get you there in fifteen seconds.

Is there a specific way of listening to music that causes this relaxation response?

There are several. One is just to have appropriate music in the background, where it can work at a subliminal level. You don't even have to be aware that it is playing, though it will change the entire atmosphere of a room. The very first field test of some of my music was in the waiting room of a doctor with whom I wanted to do some research. Babies stopped crying and mothers stopped getting angry for having to wait so long... yet nobody realized the music was even on.

I also recommend that people take a little sound bath every day. Take five to twenty minutes, close your eyes, and listen to music through headphones. Or perhaps point your feet towards the speakers, to get the sound coming through the soles of the feet. The primary thing is to allow yourself to really be with the music. Let the music wash over you. Receiving such music as a gift is a wonderful way to experience the sounds. You might also sit up with your hands held with the palms open, perhaps on your lap. Remember that sounds come into the body not just through the ears but through the whole body. So if your posture is in a receptive mode, you'll receive more benefits from the music.

Do you feel music has a place within conventional medicine as well as psychology?

I do. The appropriate music can be a powerful adjunct to conventional approaches and can enhance a wide range of therapeutic modalities. Music was one of the most ancient of the healing arts. Pythagoras was using music thousands of years ago as a specific treatment for psychological treatment of psychological and physiological illnesses. What I think we're seeing today is a reestablishment of the healing potentials of music and sound. We're developing the proper tools, too, since disco music and healing are obviously mutually exclusive realities. But when you have music especially composed to be healing and uplifting, it makes sense to use it as a resource. So instead of just reaching for a pill or other chemicals, we currently have "vitamins of the airwaves," vibrations in the form of pure music.

Why do you feel music hasn't been more widely used in medicine?

There are several reasons. In the first place, the right music hasn't been available. Healing music wasn't readily available as such until 1975, which is the primary reason it hasn't been recognized in medicine. When I started my work, there was nothing in the medical literature regarding music that was designed specifically for healing and relaxation. Who would know of such potentials? Music therapists? As far as they were concerned, the only music to use was that of Bach, Beethoven, and Mozart. But none of these composers had designed their music for relaxation as such. Perhaps one movement in a four-movement symphony might be appropriate. But you would become relaxed then—Bang!—you'd be jolted by the subsequent scherzo or loud, fast passage.

When we did our first studies, we took one of my compositions and compared it to a piece by Franz Liszt, the *Liebestraum No. 3,* which studies done by music therapists had demonstrated was soothing and relaxing. We put it against my *Spectrum Suite,* and within fifteen seconds, the *Suite* produced more relaxation than Liszt got after five minutes. We looked at such variables as galvanic skin response, EEG tracings, and the balancing of acupuncture meridians and we simply found a world of difference.

Are there other factors?

Take a look at how much training physicians get in medical school on the possibilities of sound and healing. It's zero. So most doctors come into their practices with no background in music and with a mind-set that says, in effect: "If we haven't learned it in medical school, it can't be valid."

Do you foresee this situation changing?

More and more physicians are willing to experiment with anything

72 that can help the patient. These doctors realize that they aren't playing God but are merely assisting in the healing process. They have been among the first and foremost proponents of music in medicine. Dr. Norman Shealy, for instance, recognized the efficacy of music in therapy and pain rehabilitation in 1976 and he has made music a major part of his program over the years. But some physicians feel that such music is a threat to them. Somebody can listen to the tapes, they explain, and then figure they no longer have to go to the doctor's office. So if doctors perceive music to be a threat to their practice and financial well-being, that's a reason they may resist its use.

But in general, more and more physicians are realizing that most diseases—perhaps as many as eighty-five percent—are primarily psychosomatic. So if we can help the patient establish a relaxation state so the body can heal itself, physicians can begin focusing on the patients who really need care. Physicians, surgeons, dentists, and chiropractors are adding music into their work—not as a replacement, but as an adjunct to it.

What led you, personally, to begin writing healthful and spiritual music?

I really had no choice. The music got into me! I had been interested in music all of my life. My formal training took me to a certain plateau of artistic expression and technical proficiency, but it left me feeling unfulfilled at a deep, inner level. When I read about the use of sound in the ancient healing temples, lights went on inside my head. I needed to know more, so I read everything available in the field and conducted some private research. As part of my inner work with personal guidance and meditation, the music started to come through. I started hearing it in my dreams and meditations. It was clear to me that writing such music was what I was placed here to do. I thought my job was through at that point, so I made my first tape and got it out to some hospitals and scientists. But that turned out to be only the beginning.

What came next?

At the time, there was no field of New Age music. No one had considered that music could be used in such healthful ways. When I started going to record companies with the idea, they said there was no commercial potential for music that didn't have a good beat and

lyrics. So I realized that my options were limited. Either I discovered 73
how to share my music by learning business skills—a radical depar-
ture from anything I'd studied as a musician—or starve. I realized
that my calling involved working in both worlds. For me, this has
been a path with heart and it feels as though it is what I have come
here to do.

**Are there any procedures you use when you sit down to cre-
ate a piece of music for sound health?**

Definitely. The guiding axiom I've used ever since I first began my
work is "Composer, compose thyself!" In order to play and create
music for sound health, you have to be in that state yourself. That
results from a combination of general life-style and special methods.
When I have an appointment in a recording studio, I spend part of
the day before in preparation for it. On the day of the recording I per-
form some meditation or T'ai Chi and spend time out in nature, walking in the woods and sitting with the trees. I find that I have to book
the studio for the entire day just to keep extraneous vibrations out of
the room, even if I'm not recording all day. I pay so somebody else
isn't in there. I realize that the recording studio is my sound temple
and I revere it as such. When I begin recording, I do an opening affirmation and prayer that the music to be composed will be of service to
its listeners. I learned many years ago that the music comes through
me, that I am a conscious cocreator of it, a channel through which it
can manifest. I realized that it wasn't all "my" music.

Are there factors that interfere with this process?

Once, as I was on my way to the studio, somebody ran into my car
in a parking lot. I thought I had cleansed the incident from my mind
by the time I got into the studio. But when I later listened to the tape
of that day's session, even though it sounded okay, there was an over-
tone that didn't feel right. Much to my recording engineer's surprise, I
asked him to erase the tape.

**Are there ways that everyday sorts of people, people without
particular musical talents or skills, can use music for their
own spiritual enhancement?**

Definitely. Listening to the appropriate music, such as *Crystal
Suite*, will literally meditate you. Being in the presence of such music

74   and tuning into it can be marvelous. You don't have to be a musician to appreciate it. You already have your own instrument within the body, and such music will tune it up.

I also recommend singing in the shower. The hard, reflective acoustical surfaces in the bathroom enhance the voice. You don't even have to sing words. Just toning on certain vowels by hitting a low note and creating a gradual glissando to a high pitch will trigger some interesting responses in the body. It will increase energy in the body and release endorphins. Singing in the car or outside with the birds can also be great things to do. Notice that you never see birds practicing, so don't be shy about singing to them. They aren't going to be critical and they love singing along with you—especially if they are mockingbirds.

I also suggest you start thinking about reducing stressful noise in the environment. If you live near traffic and can't move, get some gentle music to use as a sound conditioner. More and more sound tracts are becoming available for meditation, and a great deal of classical music and New Age music can be used as foreground music.

Remember that music is here to be explored. Too many people today have forgotten how to simply listen to music, so give attention to the interior of what you hear, without the need to analyze what's going on. Listen to it in terms of its being an experience rather than something to be figured out. Just as we don't understand why aspirin works, neither do we know how music produces the effects it does; however, it can bring relaxation and healing into our lives, and we ought to appreciate it and use it as fully as possible for those purposes.

4 | THE COURAGE TO GRIEVE

AN INTERVIEW WITH JUDY TATELBAUM

B I O G R A P H Y

Judy Tatelbaum is an experienced psychotherapist, lecturer, and educator who has specialized in freeing people from emotional suffering. She graduated from the Simmons College of Social Work in Boston after taking her B.S. degree from Syracuse University. She then worked for several years at the Massachusetts Mental Health Center of Boston and the Payne Whitney Psychiatric Clinic of New York City. She subsequently established a private practice as a grief counselor and Gestalt therapist. Her first book, *The Courage to Grieve: Creative Living, Recovery, and Growth Through Grief*, published in 1980, was followed by *You Don't Have to Suffer: A Handbook for Moving Beyond Life's Crises*, published in 1989 (both released by Harper & Row). She lives in Carmel Valley, California, and is a frequent lecturer throughout the country.

Ever since first reading *The Courage to Grieve,* I knew I wanted to meet its author. It was the perfect book on the subject—concise, practical, and oriented to spiritual as well as psychological concerns. Two years passed before I had the opportunity to meet Judy Tatelbaum. She was traveling extensively to promote her second book and I finally caught up with her at Los Angeles International Airport. Our interview took place in unlikely surroundings, given the serious topic of our talk. Snuggled into a corner of a United Airlines lounge, we became absorbed in conversation, barely noticing the jangle of clattering dishes and the low drone of people chatting at nearby tables.

D. SCOTT ROGO: Can you explain what bereavement counseling is and what it tries to accomplish?

JUDY TATELBAUM: A bereavement counselor helps people fully express their feelings around a loss, something that may be hard to do with family and friends. When it is successful, bereavement counseling serves to help people come to terms with the experience of having someone close to them die, and helps them to recover and go on living a full life.

Of all the aspects of social work and psychology, what drew you specifically to working with the bereaved?

My brother died in an automobile accident when I was seventeen. It was a great shock. I had no previous experience with death whatsoever. Nor was there any counseling available to me. At my request, my parents sent me to a psychiatrist, but he never really talked to me about my brother's death. So my grief persisted for years until I took part in a Gestalt therapy training group with Jim Simkin, a well-known Gestalt therapist. I brought up a dream... a dream in which I was so angry I tried to drive into people. I was upset that I would have such a dream. Jim wanted to know when I had it. Now that was probably the first time I had ever admitted feeling this anger, but even then my remark was more of a casual statement than a conscious acknowledgment of my feelings, because I didn't understand them yet. Jim drew up a chair and told me to imagine that my brother was sitting in it. "Tell him you're angry at him for dying," he said. It was shocking to me. How can you be angry at a dead person? I was very frightened by the experience, but I trusted Jim completely. So I "told" my brother that I was angry at him for dying.

What was your emotional response to the exercise?

A great deal of emotion surfaced. I expressed many of the feelings I had when I was seventeen, right after my brother died; feelings of resentment, betrayal, and abandonment. For example, he had promised to teach me how to behave with boys, and I resented his not keeping his promise. Jim then asked me to say good-bye to my brother. I told him I couldn't do it. I really thought that, if I did, thunder and lightning would strike or the world would come to an end. But finally when I did manage to say good-bye, nothing happened. I was a bit disappointed and said so to Jim. His response was "How about saying: Good-bye David, hello world?" So I said those words and I looked around at the other participants sitting in a circle around me in this workshop and they were crying. I was very moved that these people had lived through this experience with me. Something really shifted within me. At that moment I finally let go of David and became part of the world. For fourteen years I hadn't done that!

That experience was instrumental not only in healing you but also in leading you into grief counseling?

Yes, it was. Reflecting back, I saw my fourteen years of grieving as tragic. I saw that people really need to talk about and have some means for letting go of their losses and that often there is not enough opportunity for them to do so in this society. People can feel very isolated and alone when they are grieving, and I knew something could be done to help them with their pain.

You've been focusing on the psychological aspects of your experience. Were there spiritual aspects to it?

After I had completed my grief over my brother with Jim Simkin in

78 1971, I moved to California and for the first time met people who believed in life after death. I had not been raised with that belief, but here in California it seemed prevalent. I was curious but not convinced. Then in 1975 I attended a conference in San Francisco on death and dying. Elisabeth Kübler-Ross told an audience of a thousand people that she had no doubt there was life after death. At that moment I clearly understood the meaning of several dreams I had experienced involving my brother. I saw them in an entirely different light.

After my brother died, I had frequent dreams in which he came to me saying he lived someplace else now... that he could come to me but I couldn't go to him. It was a place without phone books, without phones, without addresses or street numbers. I realized then that my brother was trying to tell me that he did still live somewhere but that the place wasn't like here. I had similar connections with people who have died since that time.

Why do you think people have such a difficult time with the loss of a close friend or relative?

I believe one reason is that we're not usually taught much about death. So when someone close to us dies, we're usually shocked. We don't accept death as a natural part of life. We think relationships should and will last forever. Of course that's not true, so we are bound to be deeply disappointed.

Dr. Kübler-Ross views death as having five "stages": shock, denial, bargaining, depression, and eventually acceptance. Do you believe there are similar stages to the process of grieving?

Yes, but the stages don't happen in an orderly fashion, nor do they occur in specific time periods. Sometimes a person might go through one of these stages in five minutes, only to return to it three weeks later or three months later. What I see is three stages. First there comes a period of shock during which the person is trying to adjust to the death or loss. Next comes a period of disorganization and suffering, in which the grieving person experiences all sorts of intense emotions. The third period is when the person begins to reorganize and reenter life. This period comes when the loss is no longer the focal point of the person's life. The sense of loss is still there but it becomes secondary.

Do you believe everyone grieves in the same way?

Absolutely not, I have met people who are already suffering deeply after the death of a loved one, who then suddenly go into shock when the loss hits them in a different way. I've seen people who seem organized for a period of time following a loss but who later deteriorate. In my professional work I've witnessed almost every possible variation of grieving. I think we make a serious mistake by setting a standard for how grief should be experienced. The important point to remember is that the grieving process is healthy. When the loss occurs, we need to grieve and to feel all the feelings of pain, sorrow, anger, and regret. That's what helps us recover.

The specific form of the grief process, however, is going to vary from person to person, depending on the relationship between the person and the deceased. One thing I always like to explore is how close the relationship was in the first place. More and more I'm learning that when you've loved somebody purely—when you've said and done everything there is to say and do—it is easier to let go of them. That's different from relationships where there's a lot of unfinished business, a lot unresolved. Those are the tough relationships to let go.

Aren't there some people, though, who simply don't grieve? I'm not referring to people who hide or deny their grief, but healthy people who come to terms with death easily?

Yes, a few. I once met a woman who seemed to have a great understanding and acceptance of death. When her granddaughter died in a plane crash, she felt sorrow but she didn't grieve. She told me that she views "the other side" as being better than here so the death wasn't overwhelmingly sad to her. She said she would miss her granddaughter but could not grieve for her.

Aside from such exceptional cases, there are people who don't grieve properly. You call it "unsuccessful" grief in your book *The Courage to Grieve*. Could you define this term and perhaps cite some examples?

We see unsuccessful grief when people try to be stoic. People who, in the face of a loss, try to swallow hard and "tough it out." Usually they are denying sadness and anger, and are suffering in some ways. They may be detached from their lives, withdrawn from loved ones, or

80 angry at everything, but they never connect these feelings with their loss.

I remember seeing a forty-year-old woman who appeared almost twice her age after her husband died. Her entire body had rigidified. She began to slump and she developed a hump on her back. She was frozen with grief and she wouldn't talk about it. These are people who might have heart attacks six months after their losses, because they haven't dealt with their feelings. I'm very concerned with the physical aspects of grief. When people don't express their feelings, they sometimes become ill.

I was just about to ask whether grief can affect a person physically as well as emotionally.

During the process of grieving, you can feel physically terrible. You can have aches and pains, you can get the flu, and you feel depleted. The body is often affected by a loss, especially when the loss is that of a spouse, lover, or child. It feels like the body has been ravaged in some way. People who have gone through a severe illness with their beloved sometimes develop that person's symptoms temporarily. I've seen this, for example, in partners where one person has died from AIDS. The other person begins to develop similar symptoms, even though he or she is not ill. It is a sympathetic reaction. I've heard horrendous stories of people who think they have cancer or heart disease after somebody they love had died. We identify with the people we love.

Could you talk a little more about specific kinds of unsuccessful grief?

One form is the overexaggerated These people make memorials or shrines to the people they've lost. I wrote about one person in *The Courage to Grieve* who created a shrine to her deceased husband. A similar reaction is to leave the deceased person's room identical to the way it was while the person lived, years after the death. Unsuccessful grief is often grief that extends too long in time. For me, too long is beyond a year or two. Generally, people need to be completing the grieving process within that period of time.

What would you suggest people do about incomplete or unsuccessful grief?

People need to realize they are in trouble and get help. I have been very concerned particularly about how long many people spend grieving, such as taking years to recover from a loss. This is one of the things that led me to write my new book, *You Don't Have to Suffer*, to show people the ways we keep ourselves stuck and the ways out of suffering. I think we have much more choice about how and how long we grieve than we often think we do. I am concerned that one of the main things that keeps us stuck is that we feel like victims of our losses and our painful life experiences. There is no power in that. My new book is intended to help free people from feeling like victims.

If a person is trying to deal with grief and is having a difficult time working through it, what resources are available to him or her?

Nowadays there are bereavement groups. People feel very isolated when they are grieving. They feel all alone, as though they are the only ones ever to go through this ordeal. They can't imagine that anybody else would understand. But in a bereavement group you find companions, *compadres*, people who *do* know what you are going through. There are groups for people who have lost friends or relatives to AIDS or cancer. There are groups for people who have lost children, and support groups for widows and for widowers. This is the day and age of the support group, and that's probably one of the most powerful tools out there. You can see other people recovering, and you know you too can recover.

A second thing a person can do is seek counseling. You need to know, however, that not all counselors are good with grief work. A hospice is a good resource for referrals. You can seek counsel from a minister or someone else in your church. It doesn't have to be a trained therapist. Sometimes someone else who has grieved can give enormous understanding. This is part of the power of such groups as the Widowed Person's Service. When you are vulnerable, it may be hard to evaluate the person you're talking to. What you want is someone who will really be there for you and your feelings, who can help you express your pain and who can tolerate your pain with you. If you feel better afterwards, that's a good way to know whether talking has been of use to you.

Are there any other resources available to grieving persons?

82   There's a technique I describe in both of my books which is a way literally to say good-bye. You can do this procedure alone, with somebody sitting with you, or with a therapist.

How is it done?

It's similar to the chair technique I used to say good-bye to my brother. Imagine you are placing the departed person in a chair facing you. Carry out the dialogue with that person until some sort of resolution of any unfinished business is reached. Begin by sharing out loud whatever comes to mind, such as "I'm angry" or "I'm hurt" or "I'm sorry." Previously hidden feelings may rush forth after your opening statements. This is the time to say whatever you feel. If you suspect you still have unexpressed feelings in a particular area, keep repeating what you have already expressed, until the things you need to say emerge.

Often a central part of the process of finishing with grief is acknowledging that the person is truly gone. If we are denying the death, we need to confront the reality of it. Admitting the death can be a relief. Understanding and finishing with loss hinges on our admitting what we lost. Knowing precisely what is gone enables us to grieve and perhaps fill that gap in the future.

So far we've been discussing some psychological aspects of loss, and I'd like to turn now to the spiritual aspects of grief work. What do you feel are the potentials for spiritual growth through the grief process?

For many people, the experience of loss serves as an opening to their spirituality. My brother's death served that purpose for me, though several years passed before I had the spiritual experience that resulted from his death. But I know his death was instrumental in leading me to grow spiritually, and I've seen this pattern over and over again in other people.

One awareness I gained, for example, was that life goes on beyond death. Recently I was talking to a group of about three hundred people who were either going through grief themselves or working with the bereaved. For the first time in a public situation I talked about my belief in life after death and cited some things that have happened involving my own parents. They died just a few years ago and I've been having a very strong sense of connectedness with them. To my amazement, many people approached me afterwards and thanked me for opening them up to the possibility of life after death. But not everybody is able to accept this possibility. For example, my mother died before my father and I talked to him endlessly about the experiences I was having with her in dreams, trying to let him know that he was going to be with her again. He was so bereft that he didn't believe me. I couldn't get the message across. Yet when he died, he was with me almost immediately.

What was that like?

One experience that stands out happened a few weeks after my father died. A message came to me—I had a pad of paper handy and I wrote the message down. What I wrote started out: "Dear Judy, we don't want you to worry." It was a letter from my father telling me he didn't want me to worry about the new responsibilities I had since he died. (I've had to deal with some financial matters.) It was a long letter saying that he and my mother were not monitoring my life. They wanted me to feel free. The end of the letter said they had one request: that I enjoy life. It was a very beautiful experience.

Not everyone dreams about their departed relatives or friends, or feels a sense of connectedness with them. But I encourage grieving people to ask for that connectedness... to literally ask that the deceased person give them a sign. Some do. Some people have even had visions of the deceased person. I've never had such an experience, so I don't know what it's like. We don't receive experiences we aren't prepared for or can't handle. I would probably think I was crazy if I saw a vision, so I never had one! But dream contacts are very comfortable for me since I've always been very involved in my own dream life. So to encounter my deceased people in dreams seems very natural to me. Other people meditate and have a sense of talking with the people they love.

But even if you have never had a connectedness with your departed loved ones, you can still believe and know they live on. Even if you don't know where they are or what they're doing, they are forever. You can love people forever. I think of our dead as being long-distance relationships.

Doesn't this result in a prolonged period of grieving?

The biggest problem with grief is that we like to think the best testimonial is the way we grieve—how much and how long we grieve.
But that's not a great testimonial. I say that the best testimonial to our
deceased relatives is in how we live. This I think is the most important message I have to give people: not to confuse how much we love
with how much we grieve.

**You were engaged in the work that led to *The Courage to
Grieve* some ten years ago. So as we conclude, I'm wondering
where your work in bereavement counseling has taken you.
Where did it lead in your personal and professional life?**

After I wrote that book, eight people in my life died. I needed a
new set of tools to help me. One of the things I said earlier is that it
takes a year to mourn. But if I took a year for each of those eight people, I'd be mourning for eight years. When my mother was dying, she
told me she didn't want me to cry a lot when she died. I said I
couldn't promise not to. She said, "Cry a little, but don't spend too
much time on it." She opened up the possibility for me of not suffering, and I found that I was OK within two weeks of her death. When
my father was dying several months later, one day he told me how
much he hated still being alive and then I knew he didn't want to be
alive for me. I wanted him to know I would be OK. I didn't want to
lose him, but I would be all right. My father died three days later.

How did this affect your professional life?

Suddenly I had no family and an entirely new life to confront—a
life without my parents. In order to manage myself during that time, I
started writing, because writing is my favorite thing to do—it's therapeutic and clearing. My new book tried to show that we have some
choice over how much we grieve or suffer over any of life's events...
that we can be in charge of our emotional experiences instead of
being their victims. Clearly my life has been touched in the sense
that I've suffered a lot of loss. How not to be a victim of such experiences and how to take life on as a challenge instead of a predicament
is my current commitment. I've moved beyond doing individual counseling and I'm traveling around the country lecturing to get this message across.

**In essence then, what would be the most important lesson
you've been trying to teach people?**

That we can recover from anything that befalls us. Suffering is really the prolonging of our hurts. If only we had been raised to know that hurt is natural. Then life's hurts wouldn't be so painful, and we would recover more easily. We wouldn't be so afraid to live and love. We often say in the face of a crisis that we will never get over it, and such a statement can become a self-fulfilling prophecy. I think we need to learn to say, "I will get over it," and make that true in our lives. I promised my father that I would be OK when he died, a promise that I made with no certainty. I said it to reassure him, but it was a promise that I wanted to make true for me too. It worked as a very powerful stepping stone to my recovering from losing him.

We need to understand that sometimes life is going to hurt. Sometimes people are going to hurt us or leave us or disappoint us. Our bodies will hurt and let us down sometimes too. We can't avoid the fact that life will have its ups and downs for every one of us. We need to cry about our hurts and get all our feelings out—be it sadness or anger or regret or whatever we feel—and then let it all go. The important thing is to live today, free of past pains and sorrows, alive to whatever today has to offer. My commitment is to help people know they can have rich and satisfying lives today no matter what has happened before.

5 | EXPLORING THE CREATIVE MIND

A VISIT WITH DENNIS WILLARD

CREATIVITY.

It's a strange phenomenon since everyone possesses the skill, even though conventional psychology barely understands it. The early Freudians were not very interested in the subject except in terms of sublimated sexuality. It wasn't until the post–World War II days, in fact, that psychology came to respect and research the subject. This surge of interest in creativity came only when psychology began to explore our inner potentials, not simply our inner demons.

Only a few bold psychologists studied the creative process before the Second World War, but even their approaches were predominantly behavioristic. Probably the most notable research was conducted by Dr. Lewis M. Terman, a psychologist at Stanford University, who began studying gifted children in the 1920s. Dr. Terman was fascinated by the popular belief that gifted children lose their capabilities when they mature. So he followed several such children for thirty years, finding that creative youngsters usually grow into creative adults. Even more fascinating was the psychologist's finding that their early scholastic successes were matched by good social adjustment, general health, and athletic skills. Dr. Terman's studies (which culminated in the 1950s) did much to disprove the conception that creative people are nerdlike, social hermits — a stereotype often popularized by many Hollywood "teen" movies and TV programs.

Of course, creativity is not the same thing as simple intelligence, so contemporary psychology has special tests to determine each person's creative potentials. These tests have demonstrated that creativity is not specifically linked to IQ, but correlates with a person's sense of humor and his/her unconventional career choices.

But such studies have certain limitations, since they tell us relatively little about the *way* gifted people think and create. In order to map the precise cartography of the creative process, we have to start looking at creative people while they work. This was the opportunity I had in April 1988 when I visited Dennis Willard in Santa Rosa, California. Santa Rosa is a scenic little community located in northern California some sixty miles from San Francisco.

But just who is Dennis Willard? Chances are that every time you operate a computer you're using something he originally developed — including the floppy disk.

Born in a small Kansas town some sixty years ago, Dennis Willard was an exceptional person even in early childhood. He grew up in his father's machine shop, where his interest in electronics and gadgetry was first sparked. The precocious youth built a one-tube radio set (without supervision) when he was seven. From that relatively simple start he went on to invent a remote-sensing burglar detector and, during his freshman year in college, a working computer.

Despite these impressive credits, young Dennis was anything but a social misfit. He was popular in high school, studied the piano, triumphed in athletics, and excelled on the dance floor!

When he entered the University of Kansas, Dennis Willard was bound and determined to become a computer engineer... an intriguing goal since computer technology was in its infancy and nobody there could help him. But he talked the Dean into allowing him to study electronics, mechanical engineering, and mathematics in order to prepare himself. When his dedication and talents became obvious the Dean gave him some space in the engineering building. It was 1946 and that's when Willard built his first computer with vacuum tubes and pinball machine relays that he had scrounged up.

"It had rather poor computational ability," he would later explain. "But it was good at playing simple games — such as tic-tac-toe."

Several years later in New York, Willard would meet with the founder of IBM, Thomas J. Watson, Sr. His response to Willard's first-generation computer was hardly enthusiastic.

"Well, it probably was a good product for a young man to do so that he could learn something," he told the young inventor. "But you

88   should have designed it to do something else. There will never be a market for a computer that plays games with people."

So much for foresight!

Dennis Willard's career received its first important impetus in 1949 when the editor of *The Kansas Engineer* (published by the university) invited him to contribute an article on computers. When it was published several months later, the Dean sent copies to several important business executives in the United States. The result was that the University of Kansas student was invited to meet with IBM and began his long employment with them. He was immediately placed in the company's Advanced Engineering Program, where he received intensive training before upper-level management bid for his services. Willard worked first in production engineering and then went on to management positions. He subsequently became IBM's Security Officer, where he developed a special information retrieval system for retrieving classified documents — a system later used by the United States Air Force. His next break came in 1952 when he was promoted to Project Engineer and set up a technical publications operation for IBM.

During these productive years, Willard was busy with his first love: his penchant for creating and developing inventions. IBM was impressed enough to give him a $200,000 budget in 1954 to conduct exploratory research on product development.

"This was great fun," Willard would later explain. "I developed a large analog computer, programmable power supplies, invented the first digital electro-optical circuits, and did the electronics design for high-speed computer printers until the advent of laser printers."

But despite the "fun," Willard was constantly annoyed by IBM's chintzy salary and decided to change jobs. It was this plan that spearheaded him into the fascinating career of technological problem solving.

While the busy inventor was growing disenchanted with IBM, a fellow employee named Rey Johnson was urging the company to set up a research laboratory in San Jose, California. IBM was trying to develop a disk file storage device — later to be called the RAMAC — but couldn't get it to function reliably. Operations were eventually set up in California and IBM's engineers started competing to relocate to the Golden State. It was during this time that Willard submitted his resignation, which caused the company to panic. Since they desperately wanted to keep him, they began searching for projects to keep up his interest. Rey Johnson was called upon to talk with him, and the result was a job offer in California to troubleshoot the RAMAC. Willard found that the engineers working on the project were great theoreticians but lacked practical experience with computers. There were countless problems with the RAMAC but Willard eventually solved each of them.

From his work on the RAMAC, the *Wunderkind* engineer proceeded to develop a greater capacity file and a high-speed million-character file. The result was that Willard invented the precursor to the floppy disk and the linear voice coil motor still used for high-performance disk files.

It was both ironic and unfortunate, though, that the million-character file wasn't successful for IBM. The invention was too sophisticated for its existing computer systems and ended up being discarded.

Despite his rich and rewarding work for IBM, Willard was forced to play office politics while conducting his research, which prompted him to finally leave IBM. His next position was with Ampex in 1960, where he helped the company with its computer development programs—though in 1961 he received some belated recognition from IBM. The company voted him its outstanding inventor and sent him a check for one thousand dollars. It seemed like a small reward for someone who'd made millions for them.

Willard's career with Ampex was no less productive than his IBM tenure, and he constantly impressed his employers with his troubleshooting abilities. This skill became the inventor's personal trademark — i.e., taking the inventions of his coworkers, isolating problems with the systems, and subsequently solving them. He eventually embarked on a long-term program to develop several high-performance computers. These new systems used integrated circuitry instead of transistors. These computers also employed disk files and became the first monolithic integrated computers on the market. Willard's work with the series was profitable enough for him to organize his own Willard Laboratories in the 1960s, where he worked on contract for such companies as Burroughs, McDonnell-Douglas, and Kaiser Aerospace and Electronics. He eventually sold the company in 1972 to work more independently.

Dennis Willard is today a busy inventor holding forth in his private laboratory and workshop in Santa Rosa. He is currently occu-

90   pied with some fifty projects ranging from a revolutionary hearing aid to perfecting a machine to make sure dates are pitted properly. When he's not puttering around in his workshop, he designs and builds furniture and writes religious songs.

I knew a great deal about Dennis Willard's background even before I flew to Santa Rosa to meet him personally. Based on some biographical material and published profiles I had read, I was feeling pretty intimidated while making the flight from Los Angeles. I nearly flunked "shop" classes in secondary school, and still haven't figured out how to preprogram my VCR. And I was supposed to be interviewing an electronics/computer whiz?

When I finally arrived in Santa Rosa, I was immediately put at ease by Dennis — who greeted me at the hotel where the Santa Rosa bus from San Francisco terminates. His folksy demeanor and friendly handshake indicated that he was eager to share his thoughts with me. I warned him that electronics and technical subjects were my nemesis, but he didn't seem to mind and immediately drove us to his workshop, conveniently nestled in the hills of scenic Sonoma County near his home.

"I made it look like a barn so the neighbors wouldn't know what I'm up to," he said when the short trip ended. The remark puzzled me because I couldn't see any neighbors!

Dennis wanted to show me his private lab, but walking through it brought back uneasy memories of my junior high school years. Remember the shop building where classrooms for metal work, carpentry, plastics, and other crafts stood side by side? Recalling that building will give you a rough feeling for Dennis Willard's private workshop. With floors cluttered with bent nails, sawdust, and discarded wiring, the laboratory consists of several rooms devoted to such crafts as electronics, carpentry, and a storeroom filled with every conceivable nut and bolt. I could only marvel at my host's obvious talent for such a wide variety of skills.

But my real reason for coming to Santa Rosa was to explore the inner workings of Willard's mind. What *process* lies behind such a genius's creative intellect?

Later that morning, we drove over to Willard's large but comfortable home. While we sat in his living room, I asked the inventor my first question. Why did he feel he was so incredibly creative?

I think my host was surprised by the inquiry.

"I think I'm creative because I've created a lot of things," he replied. Before continuing he lit a cigarette. "Performance is a good judge of a person's capabilities."

It seemed to me that Willard probably misunderstood my question, since I was predominantly interested in the psychological factor *behind* his creativity.

"I think that it's basically a matter of practice," he continued during our talk. "If a person is interested in playing a musical instrument of some kind, he practices and practices and practices. That person may not become a virtuoso, but he or she will become pretty good at a musical instrument, even if they don't have any formal training. So creativity is partly a matter of learning informally by practice. But most of my creative work is done by sitting in a chair."

This last remark really sparked my interest since it stretched into the heart of the creative sense.

Psychologists have learned that two different processes lie behind creativity. When a creative person is presented with a problem — such as a device that doesn't function properly—there usually are only limited ways to solve it. The first form of creativity is merely to systematically implement these solutions in insightful ways until the proper solution is reached. But there is a second form of creativity which is more mysterious, for it relies upon breakthroughs from the subconscious, which often "knows" the solution long before the conscious mind stumbles upon it. These creative breakthroughs often come when the inventor has entered into a special, inwardly focused state of mind—such as dreaming or while meditating. The most famous of these experiences was reported by Elias Howe (1819–1867) and concerns his invention of the sewing machine. The East Coast inventor had been fighting with its development for years until he had a strange nightmare. Some savages had captured him and commanded him to finish his invention. The troubled sleeper noticed in the dream that his captors' spears *had eyeholes near their points.* When he later stirred from his slumber, he realized that his unconscious mind had presented him with the solution to his problem.

This type of "Eureka" experience emerges from the four-stage process of creative problem solving first identified in 1926 by Graham Wallis in his book *The Art of Thought.* Based on considerable research, Wallis gradually determined that most inventors rely upon a

92 predictable series of stages while being creative. During the first stage he studies his problem from every conceivable perspective. This stage is followed by an "incubation" period, during which the information merely sits in the subliminal mind. The solution to the problem will sometimes suddenly emerge from the subconscious in rough form—called "the illumination"—and then the solution is refined and experimentally tested.

Dennis Willard's creative process seems to follow this well-known pattern.

"The key thing," he explained to me, "is that when a company comes to me with a problem, I don't call it a problem. I call it a situation. Calling it a problem is like trying to eat a watermelon in a single gulp. You have to break down the situation into subproblems that can be solved."

Willard explained that he first studies the "situation" by collecting every piece of information possibly bearing on it. (This is a phase of the creative process which Graham Wallis called the preparatory stage.) My host illustrated his point by referring to a problem that has recently occupied his thoughts—i.e., developing a method for better testing the ripeness of pears. He tackled the problem by learning past testing procedures and then pondering the situation's central issue: "What's the difference between a ripe pear and a green pear." This information gathering process resulted in his wondering if testing the electrical impedance of the fruit's density would work. When he realized this key to the situation, Willard merely had to design a method for evaluating it.

But sometimes this simple trial-and-error strategy doesn't work and Willard relies on other stages of the creative process. Unlike some inventors, however, he has learned to tap directly into the source of his creativity by deliberately placing himself in a special mental state. This form of problem solving harks back to his earlier comment that he works best in a chair, when he just sits and thinks.

"Let's say that I'm by myself," he told me. "By the time I've gathered as much information as I can about the situation, it's a matter of centering myself and using both sides of my brain—not merely the right or left side—and reaching out to the Supermind."

I had to interrupt my host at this point. "What procedure lies behind this sort of contact?" I asked.

"I go through a meditation process," he replied. Then he suggested that we run through the process together.

Willard began by asking me to rest back on his couch and instructed me to close my eyes.

"Think of your brain as a receiving set for a great computer," he began. He spoke with the intonations of a hypnotist. "Think of the neuron chains in your brain and spine as being part of the tuning system for this great computer, which has infinite intelligence. Be aware of both sides of your brain and the center, and be aware of the flow of energy that runs from the center down through the spine. Simply tune in to the information process that is available to you and to me. Feel the energy come in."

Willard interrupted the procedure to explain that, when the energy enters the brain, the experience causes tingling sensations in the temples.

"When that occurs, it's just necessary to ask questions and answers will flow into your mind," he continued. "But you have to remain centered and you may have to ask the questions several times to really understand what the answer is, which can come in the form of words, symbols, or images."

My host ended the exercise with the concise remark, "That's all there is to it."

While experiencing this procedure, I couldn't help but think back to my interview with Dr. Janet Quinn, which appears later in this book. She, too, places emphasis on becoming "centered" while performing therapeutic touch, even though she couldn't easily explain the state. She suggested to me that the practitioner simply "knows" when he/she finally experiences it. It struck me that Willard has learned to enter a similar state, in which the potentials of the subconscious mind instantly emerge into consciousness. The procedures Willard had evolved also seem consistent with the second and third phases of Graham Wallis's model of creativity. It struck me that during his meditations, Willard speeds up the incubation phase of problem solving before receiving the illumination. Dennis Willard has, however, developed a different model to explain the source of his creative genius. He believes his creativity comes when he taps into the "Supermind."

The subject of the Supermind comes up often in talks with the

94 inventor, who conceptualizes it as *the* source of infinite information. While he speaks of this intelligence in terms of a computer, other people might simply call it God. Willard traced the development of his cosmological model back to a time when he was working with a neurosurgeon in Santa Rosa.

Since obvious similarities exist between the brain and a computer, the two professionals began swapping information. One day they were discussing the inner workings of the brain. Willard was interested in determining the process behind thought itself, so they began calculating the number of the brain's neurons. Next they subtracted the number of neurons it takes to regulate the body, its perceptions, movement, involuntary functions, and the like. While they knew that (theoretically) the brain doesn't have enough neurons to encode and explain memory, they were surprised that there weren't even enough leftover cells for thinking!

It eventually dawned on the inventor that the "mind" is something different from the brain.

"The mind does not have a one-to-one relationship with the brain," he told me. "So how do we think? That's when I started thinking about there being a Guiding Intelligence that we communicate with unconsciously."

Based on this germinal realization, Willard began to think of the mind/brain in terms of a "smart" computer terminal. He conceptualizes the brain as a computer terminal with only local computational capacities. Such terminals are fine, but they can't handle extremely complicated manipulations.

"But it you connect it by a cable to a central processor with enormous memory and power," he continued, "the terminal suddenly has enormous intelligence and potential... even if you don't know its been hooked up."

Willard believes that each of us represents a "smart" terminal inherently linked to the Supermind, existing somewhere else in the universe. While we take charge of our immediate thinking, he believes that our higher insights and creativity emanate directly from the Supermind. This cosmic source is both a creative intelligence and an impersonal reservoir of potential information, with each aspect linked to every person on Earth.

My host's cosmological scheme was provocative, but I had certain problems with it. So I asked him why this Supermind couldn't merely be his own unconscious mind. Why couldn't his insights and inventions be the products of his own cerebrations?

"If you delve into the Supermind model," he replied, "it can explain how two people can invent the same thing at the same time, four hundred miles apart."

It was obvious that Willard was speaking from personal experience. When he had originally finished perfecting the RAMAC for IBM, he and some fellow technicians began work on a billion-character file and a high-speed million-character file. Such a file storage system would easily outperform their own RAMAC, and their talks led them to suggest the use of a drum with a magnetic card wrapped around it for high-speed reading. This design was later developed into the IBM Data Cell. But by a quirk of synchronicity, an engineer employed by a rival company developed the same process that same week. The close timing was clear from the disclosure documents filed for both processes.

I countered by suggesting that such simultaneous inventions could be explained rationally. I pointed out that, given the state of contemporary technology, it isn't unusual for two people to develop similar insights for a machine's logical evolution.

But my host readily countered my position by explaining that some of these simultaneous insights were not logical extensions from the existing technology. They seemed to represent quantum leaps of insights by the inventors.

Discussing cosmology has certain benefits and limitations, so I decided to change the conversation to a second subject dear to Dennis Willard. It was clear that he doesn't consider himself different from most people, since he posits that creativity is each person's birthright. This is a viewpoint widely respected in humanistic psychology, the psychology of personal growth first conceptualized by Dr. Abraham Maslow. (Maslow presented his doctrines in his celebrated book *Toward a Psychology of Being,* first published in 1962.) The writings and theories of the New York psychologist helped to godfather the human potentials movement of the 1960s and 1970s. That creativity is each person's personal potential was emphasized, in turn, by Dr. Carl Rogers, certainly one of the most influential psychologists of modern times. Rogers sums up his position in the following famous passage from his *On Becoming a Person:*

The action of the child inventing a new game with his playmates; Einstein formulating a theory of relativity; the housewife devising a new sauce for the meat; a young author writing his first novel; all of these are, in terms of our definition, creative, and there is no attempt to set them in some order of more or less creative.

Dennis Willard shares this general viewpoint and believes that people can *learn* to be creative. His four-stage procedure works best in a group setting, but can be reworked for a person's individual use. (Before leaving IBM he taught workshops on creativity for his fellow employees, which often focused on creative problem solving.)

Learning to be creative, Willard believes, begins by taking a situation and evaluating it systematically. The first two steps of the process set the stage for the group's creativity:

Step 1. Describe the situation and any information bearing on it.

Step 2. Define the specific component problems that have resulted in the situation and their causes.

The third phase in his model for creative problem solving is old-fashioned brainstorming. The group, or the person confronting a problem, should uninhibit his/her/their mind(s) and suggest every conceivable solution—even if they sound impractical or unlikely. No thoughts on the problem or situation should be self-censored or censored by the other group members. These suggested solutions should be written down on a piece of paper or on a blackboard.

"This approach," concludes the inventor, "gives people a way to practice creativity."

When these solutions have been outlined, then the group can evaluate them and find *the* solution to their problem.

Willard also believes that such a procedure can help children become creative. Parents should encourage their children to think up solutions to their own problems, he suggests, even if these solutions don't work. The important thing is to teach them that it is OK to think up wild solutions to their problems and not self-censor their thinking or stifle their creativity.

Dennis Willard's life has been both a scientific and spiritual journey, a profound odyssey by which he has tried to understand the universe and his personal place in it. It was while developing his cosmological scheme that he first read Ernest Holmes's philosophy in 1973. After wrestling so long trying to understand life, reading *Science of Mind* teachings struck a responsive chord. When he took up an invitation to attend a Church of Religious Science service, he further realized how close his own philosophy matched that of its founder. The inventor realized he had reached his spiritual home and later helped found a Church of Religious Science in nearby Windsor, California.

Everyone from top-ranking scientists to writers and poets have tried to understand the creative sense, and Dennis Willard is little different from them. Reams upon reams of studies have been executed by psychologists and books on the subject seem to proliferate. But in the final run, it's doubtful whether psychology understands *why* some people remain creative throughout their lives. Perhaps the best "explanation" for creativity was offered by the late Arthur Koestler, certainly one of this century's literary giants. He discussed creativity in 1946 in his book *The Act of Creation,* where he states that "discovery often means simply the uncovering of something which has always been there but was hidden from the eye by the blinkers of habit."

It didn't take me long to realize that Dennis Willard cast off his blinkers years ago, and is currently challenging each of us to do likewise.

PART II. | WAYS TO SPIRITUAL GROWTH

6 | THE SPIRITUAL WORLD OF CHILDREN

AN INTERVIEW WITH KEITH HARARY, PH.D.

BIOGRAPHY

Keith Harary, Ph.D., is research director of the Institute for Advanced Psychology in San Francisco. He is a clinical counselor and experimental psychologist with over seventeen years of experience in advanced psychological research. He has published more than thirty articles on his work and is the joint author of *The Mind Race*, published in eleven countries. He has also cowritten two short books, *Have an Out-of-Body Experience in 30 Days* and *Lucid Dreams in 30 Days*. In 1983 he accepted an invitation to address the Soviet Academy of Sciences on his research. In 1984, he organized and chaired the first national conference on The Psychology of Psychic Experiences at Esalen Institute. He has given dozens of lectures for scientific and educational organizations in the United States, Canada, and Europe, including the Association for Humanistic Psychology, Stanford University, and the Smithsonian Institution.

O ne of the joys of interviewing people is letting them focus on subjects they don't often get to discuss in public. I first met Keith Harary in 1973 when we both worked at the Psychical Research Foundation in Durham, North Carolina. It was my first position with a parapsychology laboratory and Keith, then a Duke undergraduate, was taking part in research on the out-of-body experience. Not only could he induce the experience at will, but he was proficient at designing research on the subject. Keith has lived his entire career "in the shadows," so to speak, of his contributions to the scientific study of the out-of-body experience. But closer to his heart is an even more personal matter—the problems that children face, just as he once did, when they grow up psychic and "different" from other people. Keith was pleased that I wanted to focus on this subject for this interview, and he discussed how these problems could be overcome.

The interview took place across a small kitchen table in the apartment Keith and his wife then rented. This is a traditional setting when old friends speak and perhaps this domestic scene set the stage for the soul-searching Keith had to do.

D. SCOTT ROGO: Do you believe children experience a naturally rich spiritual life? In other words, because of their youth, are children more intuitively linked with the universe than we are?

KEITH HARARY: I think it's difficult to generalize about all children. By the time you can ask children about their intuitive perceptions of the world, they've usually been so enculturated that they're busier fulfilling their sex roles. They're too engaged in the culturally determined activities of growing up—engaged in meeting the expectations of their peers, parents, and teachers. So it's rather difficult to figure out what their original state was. Despite these problems, some children seem to experience a very close affinity for nature, a kind of sensitivity to the world around them merging on the mystical. But if a little boy feels that way in this culture he's apt to get such feelings beaten out of him very quickly. Such a child will have to fight very hard to maintain that sort of sensitivity in the face of cultural forces that work to make him tough and insensitive.

I know that a lot of your interest in the transpersonal and psychic experiences of childhood is based on your own experiences as a child.

Yes, but not just my own. It's also based on the experiences of other children I knew.

What kinds of experiences?

In my very early childhood, for instance, I had a close friend who was terminally ill. We used to—believe it or not, since we were just little kids—talk a lot about a sort of feeling of "connectedness" we had with nature, and what realities existed behind the immediate reality of the world in front of us. We weren't thinking about that in an occult sense. We were just interested in exploring the deeper side of nature.

We both knew he was going to die. That was pretty obvious, but it didn't seem to frighten him that he was dying. He went through the kind of anxieties you experience whenever you face a new adventure in life. It made him think and it made me think. We engaged in a lot of typical childhood activities such as playing games and that sort of thing, but we also spent a lot of time observing nature close up; we watched spiders, spinning webs, and birds and insects, and we studied leaves. We studied things that were right there in our environment, but which you usually don't pay much attention to. That led us to realize there was more to reality than merely the obvious. We began to feel there was something that extended beyond our everyday consensus reality.

A mystical sense of directly understanding the world?

If you want to couch it in those terms.

What other kinds of religious and spiritual experiences do children describe?

104   The trouble with using words such as *religious* and *spiritual* is that they bring up certain kinds of images for many people, who will interpret these words according to either traditional religious values or on the basis of their prior religious education. So I personally have a hard time using such words. I would prefer to ask a question such as the following: Do children have experiences, which, to them, imply that there is more to life than meets the "I"? My answer is: Definitely.

Children don't tend to label their experiences. But they often experience a sort of global connectedness with the world around them. In other words, they feel they are not separate from the rest of reality but are linked to it at some deep level and can interact directly with the world. This feeling is similar to what Freud degradingly called "magical thinking."

Will you elaborate on how these experiences relate to Freud's idea of magical thinking? Do you think they could be imaginary, especially when they are reported by children who haven't established their ego boundaries?

Sometimes children have the idea that if they think about something in a certain way, maybe their thoughts can influence the world—in other words, they might make something happen in the world. We grow up being told that's silly and we're not supposed to think that way. We should grow out of it. That's the traditional Freudian line.

But who is to say there isn't some connection between your thoughts and the experiences you have in the world around you? Many philosophers believe this to be true, and that idea serves as the basis for much New Thought philosophy. Psi researchers—parapsychologists—have experimentally demonstrated that the mind can directly interact with the world and perceive information at a distance, through time, or from mind to mind when this information is blocked from "ordinary" perception or analytic inference. For all we know, we might be intuitively responding to one another's thoughts on a regular basis. If this turns out to be the case, wouldn't we say that our thoughts are directly influencing events in the world around us—as well as being influenced directly by those events on more than a simple, mundane level?

I think children often feel that sort of connection between their inner experiences and the outer world. It may not be magical thinking

but rather an expression of an understanding of how reality operates. *105*
They may experience this connectedness because they specifically
don't set up culturally determined ego boundaries between their
inner experiences and the outer world.

**Do children often tell their parents about these experiences
and feelings?**

It really depends. In the first place, when you talk about children,
you must remember that they live under all sorts of situations. Much
depends on what kind of support system the child has in the family.
In the Basque culture in Spain, for example, certain kinds of intuitive
experiences—such as feelings of connectedness with the world and
all life—are normal and expected. A child in that culture would
probably feel free to discuss them. So let's just talk about children
living specifically in Western culture.

Here in the United States there's a kind of stigma against talking
about such experiences unless the family considers "religious" or
"mystical" experiences as a normal part of their religious tradition
and heritage... which usually is not the case.

It also depends a great deal on the child's gender, as I implied earlier. If you are male and you talk about feeling a special sensitivity to
nature, you will probably worry the people around you considerably.
They will worry that you won't be tough enough to handle things
when you're a little older and have to deal with the "real" world. So if
you're a boy, you're told to go out and play with tadpoles, rocks, and
baseballs. If you are a little girl, on the other hand, it's a lot more
acceptable.

**So children don't realize that adults often can't understand
or share in their intuitive experiences?**

Correct. And what's so tragic is that this deep intuitive perception
of reality is so natural to children. When you're a child, you're discovering everything for the first time. You are discovering everything
about the world. So, for example, say you had a dream that later came
true—a precognitive dream. That might not be surprising to you... or
any more unusual than learning for the first time that tadpoles
become frogs. Children don't have inherent problems in dealing with
these sorts of experiences. The difficulties come when they see the
responses of the people around them, people who say that such things

106 aren't possible or that the child *couldn't* have such an experience.

That's interesting. So far we've been primarily discussing religious and transpersonal experiences, but you seem to be suggesting that children are prone to having what seem to be psychic experiences too.

I think *human beings* are prone to having apparent psychic experiences. When I lecture, and I've lectured all over the world, I often describe certain types of commonly reported experiences of this type. Then I ask if anybody present has had them. It's an interesting situation. A certain number of people will respond affirmatively. But when I ask how many people *haven't* had them, you'd think everyone *else* would raise their hands. One possible explanation is that many people may be reluctant to admit to the kinds of experiences they're actually having, and this reluctance may be something they learned early in life.

I'm not clear whether you're saying that children are more prone to these experiences than adults.

I don't think children are necessarily more inherently psychic or sensitive than adults. It's just that by the time you're an adult you've been taught that certain things, such as psi experiences, are impossible... and that you shouldn't admit them even to yourself. Children are more open and accepting of new experiences, but you have to get to them before they "learn" that psychic experiences are "impossible." That's when a stigma is first attached to them, and it can be very confusing for a child.

And what kinds of experiences are we actually talking about?

A wide range. We could be talking about apparent psychic experiences, such as precognitive dreams, telepathy, or a sense of knowing what other people are thinking, or what's transpiring at some distant location. But let me emphasize again that children don't label or categorize their experiences.

We've discussed what happens when children go to their parents in order to understand transpersonal and psychic experiences. But what happens when they begin their formal religious education?

Things can become very difficult! In organized religion, definite kinds of interpretations are invariably given to certain kinds of apparent psychic or transpersonal experiences. You're fed a structured interpretation. Apparent precognition is interpreted as prophecy, while other sorts of experiences are called miracles. Sometimes these experiences—which, I repeat, are natural to humankind—are placed under the direct domain of God or the devil. Of course, it depends on what kind of organized religion you're talking about. But this sort of misguided religious education may separate children from their *own* power and potential. We should be telling our children that these experiences are natural human capabilities, and we shouldn't place religious connotations on them.

What's so unfortunate is that certain kinds of apparent psychic and transpersonal experiences were probably the foundation stones upon which organized religion was based. But after religion became institutionalized, religious leaders didn't want outside "competition" from anyone who felt intuitively linked with the universe and who preferred to be independent.

An equally bad situation occurs when the religious establishment tells a child that his or her experiences are imaginary, which also happens sometimes.

What is the worst that can happen to a child who receives this kind of misguided education?

In our society, a person who is beginning to have psychic experiences has practically nowhere to turn for guidance. Children in this situation are confronted with virtually the same difficulties that confront adults who have such experiences, and they may respond in many of the same complex ways as their more mature counterparts. They are also particularly vulnerable to a number of unique personal, social, and cultural problems, including their vulnerability to cults.

How do they become vulnerable to cults?

Some people who think they've had psychic experiences—especially young people—are left with very few alternatives. More often than not, they're told to deny their experiences by their parents and teachers, and they become alienated from what might be an important aspect of their lives and experiences. This dilemma often leads people—and again, especially the young and impressionable—to join questionable religious cults. At one time I specifically counseled cult

108 defectors and learned firsthand how these groups can manipulate a person puzzled by apparent psychic experiences. Their members will probably say they share the questioner's experiences and often the "answers" that conventional religion and teachers have shirked. But, of course, the cult is being manipulative and its answers are usually extremely self-serving.

If children are having psychic or religious-type experiences and go to their parents to talk about them, how should the parents respond?

They should show some interest in the child's experiences and try to answer, nonjudgmentally, whatever questions the child might have. They could suggest, for instance, that such experiences are not aberrations or something to be treated separately from the rest of the child's experiences with the world. It's also important to be honest. Children are incredibly perceptive. They know when we adults are being straight with them, and they know when we're being dishonest. So if you don't know what your child's experiences mean, say so. You can say something like, "I'm not really sure what to make of your experiences, but that doesn't mean I don't care about you or that I think it's unimportant." You could add something like, "We can try to understand it together," and then explore the child's reaction to the experiences.

What you mustn't tell children is that their experience is bad. Don't give the child that kind of ignorant response, or say that he or she shouldn't discuss such matters.

Did you have some of these problems with your own family because of your childhood experiences?

Yes, I did, and that's not really surprising. The family is the breeding ground for enculturation. In a sense, you might say, the family represents the culture. It both reflects the values and concepts we live by, and helps perpetuate them. To the extent that there is confusion within the culture about the meaning and role of apparent psychic experiences, you can expect this confusion to appear, perhaps in a more focused and intensified fashion, within the microcosm of the family. To the extent that there are unsettled issues surrounding these experiences within the family, their role and meaning within the broader context of the culture will also remain unre-

solved. Of course, I didn't understand all of that when I was a child. *109*
My own experiences were indicative of a much larger problem.

Could you elaborate a little about the difficulties you had as a child in dealing with the way people responded to your experiences?

When you ask whether I would like to discuss those difficulties as an adult, it reminds me that I didn't want to discuss them when I was a child. When I was growing up in New York, I was expected to behave like a very traditional male. I was supposed to chew gum in a certain way, spit in a certain way, and play baseball in a certain way—even to hold a bat in a certain way that was supposed to intimidate the opposition! And you just didn't go around talking about psychic or related phenomena with anybody.

What was happening to you?

Among other things, I was having out-of-body experiences and precognitive dreams. But mostly I was having these wonderful feelings of oneness with nature, as I explained earlier. Now, while I was in this state, it would appear to be perfectly normal to function psychically—to "know" what was behind the next tree or behind the next building, or to "know" what I would see in the next town I visited, even if it was a place I'd never visited before. I would also find myself feeling in close connection with animals and at that time, I had no idea what this meant. It seemed to be a natural part of reality, and I was trying to understand these feelings in the same way I was trying to understand everything else about the world.

But the people around me thought there was something wrong with a child who wanted to sit under a tree at recess and watch blackbirds to see how they behaved and to feel a strong, intuitive connection with them. Or who liked to study ants crawling around their hills and watch them carrying their food. The people around me felt there was something wrong even with *that!* They made it emphatically clear—to the point of becoming abusive and violent—that a little boy was expected to run around with other little boys and play baseball, and not contemplate nature. Period.

Are you talking about your teachers, parents, or both?

110   Other kids, my teachers, and my parents all had negative reactions to the way I wanted to be versus what they had in mind for me. They phrased it as what was "good" for me. But my experiences weren't a sign of any kind of problem and were very positive integrating experiences in my life at the time. The difficulties came when I had to deal with other people's responses to my way of looking at and experiencing the world.

The point I'm trying to make is this: Why would you take that way of experiencing the world away from a child? What would you be offering instead? What would be better than confirming to your child that he or she is connected to all life in a very real way? What could possibly justify withdrawing such feelings from a child? What effect does it have when we continue to do that to our children? Take a look at the havoc in the world around us and the question seems to answer itself.

So I take it that this range of experiences is guiding your current work on the inner life of children.

Yes. I made a commitment when I was still a child that if I ever got through that period, and I fully intended to, the difficulties I experienced wouldn't be wasted; they would at least have meaning for me in showing how I could help other children. So my own work over the past sixteen or seventeen years has been largely about understanding certain kinds of experiences—primarily psychic functioning—to see what we can say about them... objectively, subjectively, and personally. The important thing now is to educate the public so they, in turn, can educate their children.

I guess I still feel a commitment to that friend of mine who died early in my childhood. He was terribly mistreated by other children, the same way I was. Those kids were probably mistreated themselves or they wouldn't have behaved that way. They were probably being separated, through their education in the home and in the schools, from a certain kind of sensitivity to the world in which they lived.

So what work are you engaged in right now?

I've just completed my Ph.D. in psychology... and I'm in the process of completing a book about the experience of growing up different and how a child integrates that way of looking at the world into living and surviving in this culture. It's based on my own experiences, but I think it really generalizes to other children.

I'm also coediting a clinical handbook for professionals and *111* laypeople who are concerned about how to deal with apparent psychic and transpersonal experiences. Beyond that, I'm continuing in my attempt to understand psychic abilities and other related capabilities as research director of the Institute for Advanced Psychology in San Francisco, which takes an interdisciplinary approach to understand human potential.

The more we understand about the world beyond the ordinary senses, and the more the public becomes educated, the easier it will be for the children of the future. I hope the day comes when children can talk about their apparent psychic and transpersonal experiences without being hit over the head.

7 | TRANSPERSONAL PSYCHOLOGY AND THE SPIRITUAL PATH

AN INTERVIEW WITH CHARLES T. TART, PH.D.

B　I　O　G　R　A　P　H　Y

Dr. Charles T. Tart has enjoyed an extraordinary career in psychology, encompassing research into states of consciousness, biofeedback, psychedelic drugs, hypnosis, and parapsychology. He took his B.A., M.A. and Ph.D. degrees from the University of North Carolina and is currently a full professor of psychology at the University of California, Davis. He is best known for creating the first systematic approach to understanding altered states of consciousness, conducting pioneering research into the out-of-body experience and determining if ESP can be learned. During part of his earlier career, he developed scales for evaluating hypnosis depth. Dr. Tart is also one of this country's leading experts on transpersonal psychology, the psychology of spiritual growth. Two of his books, *Altered States of Consciousness: A Book of Readings* and *Transpersonal Psychologies,* are classics in psychology. His other books include *On Being Stoned; States of Consciousness; Psi-Scientific Studies of the Psychic Realm; Waking Up: Overcoming the Obstacles to Human Potential;* and *Open Mind, Discriminating Mind.*

Interviewing Dr. Charles Tart was more like talking to an old friend than completing a journalistic assignment. I first came into contact with the psychologist back in the 1960s. He was fascinated with the study of the out-of-body experience and had just pioneered the laboratory and experimental study of the phenomenon. I had undergone the experience in high school and had written to the American Society for Psychical Research in New York, where Dr. Tart learned of my encounters and asked to meet me. I didn't realize that our meeting that day on the campus of the University of Cincinnati (where I was an undergraduate) would blossom into a twenty-five-year friendship. It was a short, rushed meeting between conference sessions in which Dr. Tart was taking part.

When we met to tape this interview, the scene was suspiciously like our first meeting. We were both attending a parapsychology convention at Sonoma State College in California. This is a wonderful campus out in the suburbs and in between sessions, we snuck over to Charley's room in the dorm to discuss transpersonal psychology, one of his many interests.

D. SCOTT ROGO: Some years ago, you published a book titled *Transpersonal Psychologies*, although the volume's working title was actually *Spiritual Psychologies*. Could you explain what transpersonal—or spiritual—psychology is?

CHARLES T. TART: Ordinarily psychology is regarded as being the study of the mind, although recently it's been defined as the study of behavior. But broadly considered, it is still the study of the mind. It concerns itself with how we think, how we solve different problems, how we develop different abilities, and how our emotions affect our thinking. Psychology studies why we behave the way we do.

But I recognized years ago that the world's great spiritual traditions contain psychological systems as well. They have lots of ideas

114 and information about classical human problems that contemporary psychology also addresses. Most people don't realize this fact because the psychology is buried inside the religion, scattered through it. So it occurred to me that if the different spiritual psychologies buried inside those systems could be extracted, it could stimulate psychologists and other people to think about their minds in new and different ways.

Can you give examples of some religions which have spiritual systems built into them?

Spiritual psychologies—psychologies that show you how to grow spiritually—can be found embedded in Sufism, in various forms of Buddhism such as Zen, within traditional yogic practices, in Christianity, in the system of observing the self and its consciousness devised by George Ivanovitch Gurdjieff, and in many others. These are examples of systems that are very psychologically oriented, even though they are presented in spiritual terms.

But do they all have certain things in common, or are they different systems entirely?

I think they do have certain essentials in common. The most important is that they do not believe what we usually consider the world of the "ordinary" to represent the limits of human nature. The "everyday" is but a small subset of what we can be. They usually go even further by saying that the ordinarily perceived world of reality is a *pathological* subset or subselection of existence, and that our true destiny is to evolve toward some higher spiritual nature. If we don't know about this nature, or if we actively interfere with our growth toward it, then we generate unhappiness or problems within a world that is fallible or "sinful," to use one word for it.

That's the primary impact of the spiritual psychologies—to let us know there are human possibilities that extend beyond the ordinary realms of everyday experience.

After the Second World War, we saw the emergence of humanistic psychology, which dubbed itself the "psychology of growth." It emphasized man's psychological potentials, and was a reaction to both behaviorism and psychoanalytic thinking, with their emphasis on the deviant behavior forced

upon us by the unconscious mind. How do the transpersonal *115*
or spiritual psychologies differ from humanistic psychology?

Humanistic psychology was a wonderful development, since it said we weren't driven solely by unconscious needs, nor were we the simple product of social conditioning. It showed that we possess important qualities such as creativity that should be studied and developed in our lives. But even though humanistic psychology was revolutionary, it still wanted to be accepted within our particular culture, so it didn't question some basic and limiting assumptions concerning our basic nature.

For example, behaviorism and psychoanalysis make it very clear that the mind is the brain. This means, of course, that when you die you're dead. There is no survival. There's no real spiritual life according to this sort of psychology, unless we use the term in a very watered-down fashion as analogous to "being authentic" or "being loving." Humanistic psychology didn't really challenge such premises, and while it taught us to know our minds and potentials better and become more loving, it didn't teach us to question the mechanistic assumptions of the Western worldview.

The transpersonal psychologies raise just these issues. They show us that experiences exist where we can go beyond ourselves, where we can transcend the purely personal. The implication is that we aren't just limited personal identities operating in a limited social world. We can view ourselves as more cosmic and more spiritual beings. The transpersonal psychologies show us that these feelings are just as real and important as other kinds of psychological experiences.

Even back at the turn of the century, there were people like William James, who was trying to build a spiritual psychology based on religious experience, as exemplified in his book *The Varieties of Religious Experience.* **And you can also examine some of the early derivatives of psychoanalysis, such as the spiritually oriented psychology of C. G. Jung, who tried to integrate psychology and religion. So in the long run, is transpersonal psychology actually inconsistent with the traditional psychologies—such as psychoanalysis and behaviorism—or is it a genuine extension of them?**

I see transpersonal psychology as an extension of conventional

116 psychology. Psychoanalysis, for example, has a great deal to teach us about the world and how our minds function within it. But as soon as you take psychoanalysis as your total worldview, you've made a serious mistake. It offers only a partial view of reality, since it overlooks the spiritual dimensions of humanity. That can get you into trouble.

You keep using the term "spiritual." Can you define more clearly what you mean? Is the term analogous to "religious"?

I deliberately use the term "spiritual" and I distinguish it from "religious." When we think of religion, we usually think of a large institution where people learn to believe prescribed doctrines, where there's a power structure, where dogmas are set, and so forth. A lot of what happens in religion can be explained in social/psychological terms, and roughly the same process occurs in any institution or within any group of people. When I say spiritual, however, I'm trying to get back to the original experience that led to the development of religion in the first place.

Let me give you an example by way of a contrast. Let's say people go to church every Sunday and come to believe certain things. The result is that they eventually act in prescribed ways. They may never have had any real experience leading them to their beliefs since they act in accordance with the ways they were raised. Some observers might even argue that such behavior has no real spiritual value. Everybody knows about Pavlov's discovery of classic conditioning in dogs—ordinarily a dog doesn't salivate if you ring a bell. But if you ring a bell repeatedly right before giving the dog some food, it will.

The issue I like to raise is this: Is the dog a good dog because he's been conditioned? Or is he a bad dog? Now that's obviously a silly question since the dog has simply gone through a mechanical conditioning process which is neither good nor bad. But it is exactly what often tends to happen in our religious life. Some people have been raised to conform to a conventional religious way of thinking and, in a sense, they've been conditioned. They have been made to feel guilty when they've done something considered—or defined as—bad and they've been punished for it. On the other hand, they've been praised when they've said the right things.

But are they really good? Or is their behavior the result of a mechanical sort of process: Some people argue, and I think there's a lot of merit to their point of view, that conditioning somebody to "good-ness" has no particular moral value. Of course, we're glad that people behave nicely, but there's no depth to their feelings or behavior.

By contrast, some people do have deep spiritual experiences. They enter into radically altered states of consciousness where they transcend their ordinary, everyday view of people and reality. These people feel they have gotten glimpses into the nature of reality, the nature of being human, the nature of God and the spiritual universe.

So you are talking about what have been traditionally called "mystical" or "ecstatic" religious experiences, where the person feels he or she has merged with God and/or the universe?

Yes. And these direct spiritual experiences produce a basis for morality, one very different from that resulting from simple conditioning.

Let me expand this point a bit. If you examine the history of world religion, you can trace each religion back to a founder. It looks as though each of these founders originally reacted to a mind-shattering vision that offered them a greater view of the world. These experiences usually came by way of meditation or some other sort of practice. The problem, though, was that the founders couldn't fully communicate their experiences to the general public. In fact, one of the primary characteristics of these sorts of experiences is that they are nearly impossible to describe in ordinary language.

So when a religion begins in this way, it can go in either of two directions. In one direction, the disciples of the founder begin to take the ordinary consciousness expressions of the founder—his teachings and interpretations—and worship them as divine truth. These teachings begin to get systematized into theology and doctrine, but the original religious experience is gone. That kind of religion tends to become shallow after a while.

The other direction occurs when the founder recognizes that ordinary language is too limited to reveal his spiritual discoveries. So this founder tries to teach a spiritual *technology,* so other people can go into the same states, to encounter similar experiences. These tend to be more experiential kinds of religions.

This is, in fact, the exciting thing about the transpersonal psychologies. You realize that you don't have to believe, or not believe, some religious tract written hundreds or thousands of years ago.

118 Techniques can be developed—whether they be meditational techniques or psychotherapeutic techniques or whatever—that lead people back to the experiential basis that gave rise to religion in the first
place.

**So one of the things that the spiritual psychologies offer that
conventional psychology does not appears to be meaning,
not simply form and structure.**

Exactly. The conventional systems of psychology, even humanistic
psychology, do not provide any satisfactory answers about the meaning of life. They teach a materialistic worldview in which the universe
is just a kind of random event with no real meaning to it. Life is considered as sort of an accident. When you project that kind of thinking
into your own life, you come to see yourself as nothing but the acci-
dental product of your genes. None of it has any meaning.

I think this sort of thinking represents a fundamental sickness in
people. What materialism has tried to substitute for us is more and
more pleasure — get a sauna, get brand X vodka like sophisticated
people do. These material things, though, do not provide any meaning
for life because the materialistic framework itself says life has no
meaning. I'm convinced from my psychological work that, in order to
be healthy, people must have a sense that the universe is meaningful,
and that they have a meaningful place within it.

Of course, some people can get involved with a conventional religion and take advantage of what it has to offer. These people are
lucky, but their luck might not hold completely. When you believe a
prescribed doctrine, you tend to become rigid, and rigidity is hard to
hold onto in a world where change is the norm. So what the spiritual
psychologies offer people is a chance to explore the transpersonal
realm for themselves. People can directly experience themselves as
entities connected with the universe. That's a lot to offer.

**But since Western psychology considers itself to be a science
and a product of the scientific method, do you think these
kinds of experiences can be scientifically and objectively
studied? Can science differentiate, for instance, between a
genuine spiritual experience and a bogus, self-delusional one?**

That's a good question. The notion that science or psychology can
make such a distinction doesn't hold up very well. But I think some

science of the future—a science that evolves with humility and curiosity—will need to look at this issue. That sort of science may be able to say more concerning the difference between a genuine and an inauthentic spiritual experience.

What can science and psychology do in the meantime?

Conventional science can explore useful issues concerning various kinds of spiritual experiences. For example, we might find that a certain kind of religious experience makes people, within a few months, feel like one of the "chosen." Such people might start treating others as though they were inferior, to be used. Now that's an observable repercussion that you can study scientifically. Perhaps you won't be able to determine whether a certain experience is real or illegitimate, but you will learn that a particular kind of religious experience has costly effects and certainly seems to contradict the universal spiritual concept that we are equal and should love each other. Scientific inquiry can therefore explore the "price tag" spiritual experiences have in terms of psychological change.

What other issues can transpersonal psychology and present-day science explore?

Science and transpersonal psychology can also explore whether there are especially efficient ways of inducing spiritual experiences. Lots of techniques exist throughout the world for inducing religious experiences — from fasting, to meditation, to dance. However, something we know from psychology is that people living in different cultures are different in many substantial ways. Their minds are structured differently, for one thing. Even within the same culture, the structure of the mind—the way people think—seems to change radically between historical periods. So the best technique for inducing spiritual experiences that was available if you were a Brahmin in India in 300 B.C. may be useless today. Perhaps transpersonal psychology can increase the efficiency of progress on the spiritual path. I think some people practice inappropriate techniques and waste their time.

Can you cite an example?

I can draw on some general impressions I have of the field. Here's one kind of example:

Some people have a certain kind of personality structure where

120 they tend to compartmentalize their experiences. For example, they only notice what's happening to them at the present moment. They isolate parts of themselves from themselves. They also tend to be withdrawn from other people. For this kind of person, being on a spiritual path that relies on meditation may present a problem. Sitting alone for long periods of time and focusing on an object of concentration could reinforce this problematic aspect of their personality.

Someone in an advisory role might want to psychologically test a person who is beginning to engage in spiritual practices. If this specific kind of personality structure was discovered, the individual could be informed that he or she runs the risk of feeling more isolated and withdrawn from other people through the practice of meditation. One could suggest, though, that these people take up something like Sufi dancing. This form of spiritual exercise involves integrating body, mind, and emotion and is conducted with other people. It would offer a corrective to this person's tendency toward too much isolation.

I dream that someday we'll develop a psychological test by which you could advise clients of the specific, most effective kind of spiritual practice for them. We're a long way from that day, but it's possible.

So as a psychologist, you're suggesting that a person should shop around for a spiritual path?

Yes. In my recent book *Waking Up,* I offer several chapters dealing with this whole question. I definitely advise people to shop around. To just "jump in" and get totally involved with the first or second path you find could be dangerous, if not wasteful. But don't shop around casually. Give some energy to a particular path. Give it a month or two to see where a given practice is leading you. You'll probably find some paths that strike you as so-so; some that turn you off; but some that offer a real "feeling of heart." When you find a spiritual path with real heart for you, you might think of making a commitment to it. See where it leads you.

What practical advice would you give someone just starting out toward the spiritual path? In other words, what things should such a person be on the lookout for? What would represent danger signals?

I don't claim to have the whole perspective, but I do look at this issue in a chapter in *Waking Up* that deals with "problems on the path."

There are two main ways you can protect yourself. One is to look out for certain signs that something unhealthy is going on in a group. No single sign may be sufficient in itself to warn you off, but if enough are present, that's bad news. For example, does a group have "secrets"? Does it conceal many of its activities from the public? It's a bad sign when a group presents one face to the public and a different one in private. Is there a feeling of elitism within the group? Do they tell you that now you are one of the "chosen"? Does the group contain spiritual clones—that is, people who copy the teacher in all sorts of ways that are irrelevant? Can you ask where the money goes? If you aren't allowed to ask that question, that's a bad sign... especially in Western culture!

And the other thing you recommend?

When you decide to follow a path that resonates for you, I suggest you go through a procedure I call the "spiritual commitment contract." This procedure is based on the psychological fact that spiritual practices won't work unless you really give some energy to them. But once you give energy to these systems, you run the risk of being changed in ways that might create real problems. This is especially true if you get involved in a so-called "cult" to use the purely negative sense of that word.

The spiritual commitment contract is a procedure whereby you sit down and write yourself a long letter. Do this just before you get involved in a spiritual group. Describe what you're like now, what you really value in life, and what you really want to achieve by trying to grow spiritually. Then you make yourself a sacred promise in this letter that you are really going to commit yourself to this group for a fixed period of time, say a year or two. That long. But you also make a sacred promise to yourself that, at the end of that time, you will separate yourself from the group for at least a month. This entails getting away from all the people involved and all their literature. This will give you the opportunity to sit down and reread your letter concerning who you were and what you really wanted. Then make as objective an evaluation as you can about what has happened during the past year or so. Have you gone in the direction you wanted? Do you want a better direction? Have you gone in a worse direction?

You should also give a copy of this letter to your best friend, and get his or her sacred promise to deliver it back to you when the end of

122   this period comes. His intercession will remind you of your promise to yourself. You'll have to get a really deep promise from your friend, though, since people often tend to change their friends when they join spiritual groups. Your best friend may decide that you've become a real creep. Or the reverse may also happen. But you will both have to remember the promise in terms of the friendship that existed when you began the involvement.

The spiritual commitment contract is a safety line by which you can pull yourself out of any group. It's not foolproof, but it's a way of letting yourself take the plunge without going too far over your head.

Finally, as a psychologist reared in the Western scientific tradition, what do you see in the future of transpersonal psychology?

Transpersonal psychology will continue becoming a diverse enterprise. Right now there are some transpersonal psychologists, for example, who have a primarily scientific interest in the spiritual. They'd like to know which spiritual realities exist in the universe and which don't; how they work and what effect they have on people. It's sort of a curiosity rather than a strong obligation driving their commitment, and that's fine. We need those psychologists.

There are other transpersonal psychologists who already have a commitment to some particular spiritual path. So their transpersonal psychology is really a subset within the wide range of transpersonal psychologies. They're into yoga, Sufism, or something like that. These people are necessary, too. But they should be clear in distinguishing themselves from those psychologists who are trying to take a more objective, scientific viewpoint.

Others have a broader view of things. They are actually fairly deeply involved in several different kinds of spiritual paths, while keeping an objective, scientific interest in what's most efficient for spiritual growth.

I think this is all going to continue to expand, because our culture has an enormous spiritual hunger, and most of this spiritual hunger is being satisfied with fast food. It seems to work for a while, but it's not very nutritious.

I'm hoping that the study of transpersonal psychology will gradually give rise to spiritual practices that are more effective and less cluttered with outdated cultural baggage. Then people can embark on the spiritual path without risking their mental health, or having serious problems during their journey.

8 SPIRITUAL HEALING IN THE CHRISTIAN TRADITION

AN INTERVIEW WITH THE REV. MORTON T. KELSEY

B I O G R A P H Y

Morton T. Kelsey is one of the best known writers on religion in the world today. Born in Depue, Illinois, he grew up in Palmerton, Pennsylvania. Graduating with honors from Washington and Lee University, he completed his theological training at the Episcopal Theological School in Cambridge, Massachusetts, and later did graduate work at the C. G. Jung Institute in Zurich, Switzerland. After ordination he became the rector of St. Luke's Episcopal Church in Monrovia, California, and subsequently joined the faculty of the University of Notre Dame. Professor Kelsey has lectured widely throughout the United States, Europe, and Asia, and has also written over twenty books. Among these are *God, Dreams and Revelation: A Christian Interpretation of Dreams; The Other Side of Silence: A Guide to Christian Meditation; Afterlife; Christianity as Psychology: The Healing Power of the Christian Message;* and *Medicine and Christian Healing.* He makes his permanent home in Gualala, California, where he is still active as a writer.

I've been reading Morton T. Kelsey's books since I was a teenager, but I never thought I would ever meet him. I can't think of any serious religious writer who has written more books on such a gamut of subjects. Rev. Kelsey's work is doubly interesting since he combines insights from both psychology and Christianity in building his case for mankind's spiritual nature.

One of my great disappointments in life is that I still haven't really met the Rev. Kelsey. When this interview was scheduled, he and his wife were in Hawaii looking after a seriously ill relative. Our talks had to be restricted to the telephone. It is difficult to describe the impression Dr. Kelsey makes when he speaks. His intonation and style of delivery remind me of an old-time preacher sermonizing. But it is a little inappropriate to describe him as an "old-timer." (Even though Dr. Kelsey is an octogenarian, every time I called Hawaii his wife explained that he was out jogging!) His literary output would put many younger writers to shame.

Dr. Kelsey pioneered bringing spiritual healing back into the church, and the occasion of this interview was the reissue of his excellent *Healing and Christianity* under the title *Psychology, Medicine and Christian Healing.*

D. SCOTT ROGO: You are probably this country's foremost writer on religion, psychology, and spiritual healing. Would you describe for us your theological and psychological background?

MORTON T. KELSEY: I'm an Episcopal minister. I originally did graduate work in philosophy before I went on to the Episcopal Divinity School in Cambridge, Massachusetts, where I graduated summa cum laude. I then became interested in psychology as I began to deal with my own problems. I found that I had been given no theological help in coming into contact with the divine, or in dealing with the depths and complexities of the human psyche. So I went into Jungian analysis and took graduate courses at Claremont College in California. Then I went to Zurich and studied at the Jung Institute for three months.

While there I had a very interesting dream in which I was building Byzantine churches. And as we talked this over at the Institute, we realized that my job was back in the church, not as an analyst but as a clergyman and theologian. My task was to integrate into the twentieth-century Western Christian Church the depth and wisdom of the great Greek thinkers of the early church. So I went back to the parish and remained there for the next fifteen years. I became licensed as a marriage, family, and child counselor in California. Then I was invited to go to the University of Notre Dame, where I helped to make Ph.D.s without having one myself!

In your recent book *Psychology, Medicine and Christian Healing*, you reprint the following citation from an article in the December 1959 issue of the *Current Medical Digest*: "Sometimes it is forgotten that medicine owes it greatest debt not to Hippocrates, but to Jesus. It was the humble Galilean who more than any other figure in history, bequeathed to the healing arts their essential meaning and spirit." Could you comment on this provocative statement?

That issue of the *Current Medical Digest* was given to me by a psychiatrist with whom I had lunch every other week for about fifteen years. The article you mention was written by someone who was a professor of medicine at Loma Linda Medical School. What the passage is saying is this: The basic attitude of modern medicine, to heal whenever healing is necessary, is basically the gift of Jesus and not of Hippocrates. Jesus is the one who gives the impetus to modern medicine, for he particularly urged that everyone who needed help should have it. The Greek world didn't give a damn about the poor. If you couldn't hire a physician, that was your tough luck!

Another interesting point is that among the Greeks, and also among the Hebrews, sickness was a sign of the displeasure of God. But Jesus gives us quite a different viewpoint. Through his teachings we see God as caring about our healing, not bringing our sickness. Jesus healed the souls, minds, and bodies of human beings because God loves us and wants us to be whole and then he also sent his disciples to do this kind of healing.

What role did the practice of healing play in early Christianity and why was it so important to the early church?

126   First of all, the ministry of Jesus involved three aspects—preaching, teaching, and healing. But it is fascinating to note that there's much more recorded about healing than about teaching and preaching! As a matter of fact, 727 verses in the four Gospels out of a total of 3,779 verses relate directly to Jesus' healing ministry. That's about the length of the entire Gospel of Mark. No other great religious leader placed that much emphasis on healing of the bodies and minds of human beings.

Secondly, Jesus brought with him a view of God as love—not the ambivalent God of the Old Testament and the Greek and pagan worlds. A completely new conception of God as caring and loving, not as vengeful, comes through the teachings and ministry of Jesus.

You state in your book that healing within conventional Christianity had its "ups and downs." Would you explain what you mean by that?

For the first glorious, powerful centuries of the early church healing continued unabated in Christian practice. Then it died out in the Western branch of Christianity. However, this ministry never ceased in the Eastern Orthodox churches. You would still find, in these churches, votive symbols of legs, arms, and hearts that are placed on the altar, after people have prayed for healing and it has been granted to them. The altars of these churches are simply covered with them. We tend to forget the rich tradition of Eastern Christianity, which has never lost the emphasis on healing that Jesus and the early church exemplified.

So these "ups and downs" occurred primarily here in the West?

Yes. Jesus' vision was lost in the West due to two or three factors. First of all, civilization collapsed. At the time of the Dark Ages in Western Europe, Byzantium or the Eastern Empire was flourishing. But in the West, life looked hopeless. Believing in healing is difficult in a collapsing culture. Then on top of this, one of the great church fathers had gout. His name was Gregory the Great [A.D. 540–604] and he wrote a book entitled *The Book of Pastoral Rule*, in which he said that God shapes us by our sicknesses and adversities into the proper kind of stones that can be built into the walls of the city of God. Thus, he appears to be favoring sickness over wellness.

Now you might be asking, what difference did this one little book make? Well, civilization came almost to a halt between 600 and 800

A.D. in the whole of Western Europe. But when Charlemagne finally began to get civilization back on track, he decreed that this book, *The Book of Pastoral Rule,* be placed in the hands of every bishop, along with the Canons of the Church and the New Testament. So Gregory the Great's attitude towards sickness gradually permeated the Western church. After that time some perfectly fascinating things happened. The church became opposed to medicine. The view was actually accepted that it was better to be sick than it was to be well! Then in 1215 A.D., the Fourth Latin Council decreed that no person try to heal anyone who hadn't been confessed first. In other words, it was better to die than to be healed without confession. Unbelievable... but true.

What factors eventually led to the current renewal of an interest in spiritual healing within Christianity?

There have always been sporadic signs of this interest. For instance, one of the signs of being a saint in the Catholic tradition, even in the Dark and Middle Ages, was that the candidate had performed healings. But the really significant development started with the work of Franz Anton Mesmer [1734–1815], who realized that the mind had a tremendous influence upon the condition of the physical body. From that basis, Phineas P. Quimby [1803–1866]—who was a pioneer mental healer in America and is considered by some people to be the originator of New Thought—got the notion that this influence of the mind on the body was a religious function. Remember that Mary Baker Eddy received her initial training under Phineas Quimby, but she went on to evolve the idea that the physical world— of which disease is a part—is not actually real, which in turn led her to believe that anything, including healing, was possible.

Quimby also believed that physical healing was possible but his approach was different. He saw healing as the result of the individual mind being in touch with Divine Mind, and he was a very successful healer. From Quimby's work came the modern realization that one main aspect of Jesus' ministry had been healing. This was a real revelation, starting from the middle of the nineteenth century. The mainline churches should be grateful to these pioneers in spiritual healing.

I'd like to turn now to your own personal involvement with spiritual healing. I take it that your specific interest in the subject was ignited by some of your personal pastoral experiences.

128   It was ignited by Agnes Sanford, who was one of the most remarkable healers within the last century. She was suffering from a depression and was healed through the laying on of hands. She became deeply interested in healing after this incident and gradually began to practice spiritual healing within her own family. Then she extended it beyond the family and began to read everything she could find. She read the New Testament and finally wrote a book called *The Healing Light*. Someone gave me a copy of it and my wife happened to pick it up one day. She found it entrancing and read it straight through. Later, she said to me that the author of the book was either crazy or a liar, or there was some truth in what she had written.

My real conversion was when, having read the book, I decided to try a version of "laying on of hands" to cure a headache my wife had. Without telling her what I was doing, I simply put my arms around her and prayed silently. Not only did her headache go away, but she had a profound religious experience which lasted for several days. That was very convincing.

Then I went back to my parish and in several cases where I felt it was impossible for someone to live, I practiced spiritual healing. Not only did they live, but they got well and were able to resume their normal lives. Then I began to search the Bible and the writings of the early church fathers. I found that in every one of the major leaders of the church up until 600 A.D., the time of Gregory the Great, healing was seen as the first fruit of having Jesus' spirit within them. The ability to heal came from the Holy Spirit and was available to everyone who embodied that spirit and consciousness.

What further evidence have you seen that spiritual healing is becoming a more significant feature of contemporary Christianity?

I've seen it in Agnes Sanford's work. I've also conducted conferences for the last thirty years on the subject. In nearly every conference there have been some quite remarkable healings.

Could you describe such a healing?

After I read Agnes Sanford's book I had a rather active hospital ministry. I was called to the hospital on one occasion some thirty years ago. I found when I got there that the people who called me really didn't want me to minister, but to recommend the most reliable

undertaker. I asked them if they minded if I prayed and they said it *129*
couldn't do any harm. The man whom they had called me about was
only forty-five years old and was in a terminal coma. I prayed for him.
The next morning I returned to find that he was still alive. For fourteen days I came in and offered prayer, morning and night. And on
the fifteenth day he was conscious and he went home and lived a normal life.

**Some theologians believe that healing should not be empha-
sized within Christianity, feeling that the Christian who isn't
healed would become discouraged with his or her religion.
How do you respond to this opinion?**

Thank you for asking me that question! In the Parish of St. Luke's
in Monrovia, California, where I first practiced a full healing ministry, we had three healing services every week. People would call us
before they went to the hospital and we would go and visit them.
During twenty years, we never had one complaint from anyone about
the healing ministry and this was a large parish. But we didn't ever
promise healing. We said that if the healing didn't come, it was our
failure, not the failure of the person to be healed.

**So in other words, in your experience people don't become
discouraged even if they don't receive healing.**

That's absolutely true. In fact, sometimes these people had
remarkable spiritual awakenings after the laying on of hands. It's
simply not true that people become discouraged, unless you specifically promise that you're going to heal somebody. But if you say, "I
am an inadequate instrument and I do the best I can," the person
doesn't become discouraged. That's a terribly important point.

**Some physical illnesses have strong emotional components
associated with them. How can spiritual healing be used to
treat not only the outer, physical but also the inner, psychological factors contributing to a person's illness?**

To answer that question, I'd like to quote Dr. Jung, from a letter he
wrote to P. W. Martin, the author of the book *Experiment in Depth*.
Martin was one of the first religious writers to see the religious significance of Jung's ideas. Jung wrote to him in 1945: "You are quite
right. The main interest of my work is not concerned with the treat-

130 ment of neuroses but rather with the approach to the numinous. But the fact is that the approach to the numinous is the real therapy and inasmuch as you attain to the numinous experiences you are released from the curse of pathology." In other words, Jung believed that our mental illness is the product of a sick civilization which has separated us from vital religious experience, from a continuous experience of God. He wrote in another place that he had never seen a case of neurosis in which the person had not been cut off from the religious experience of which all great religions of humankind speak. He'd never seen anybody truly healed until they were brought back in touch with the divine.

I personally doubt whether a person can live a wholly normal and healthy life in hopelessness, meaninglessness, and depression. The only way we're going to be sure of meaning and hope and health is to be in touch with the Spirit of God within and beyond us.

Do you believe that everyone has the power to heal?

Yes, I think everyone has the latent power to heal. Proof to validate this position can be found in studies done on babies. Pediatricians were discovering thirty-five years ago that about a third of newborn infants in an orphanage died during their first year of life and that their deaths were caused by a gradual wasting away. It occurred to these doctors that the babies needed human touch, so they brought people in merely to hold the babies. These were ordinary people who just picked up the babies and held them instead of leaving them in their cribs. In the first year, the death rate from disease dropped to ten percent. Human touch conveys love. And the love conveyed through human touch conveys the life and power of God — which are healing. Some of the most convincing books about the healing power of faith and love are not written by theologians or ministers, but by medical doctors, books like Andrew Weil's *Health and Healing* and James Lynch's *The Body's Response to Human Dialogue.*

I want to raise an important question. If spiritual healing works on a spiritual level, is it accurate to say that physical touch is absolutely essential to healing?

No. Physical touch is not essential for spiritual healing. However, it does often help the healing process.

Some metaphysical traditions teach that it is a perception of *131* **wholeness that heals and thus physical touch or any technique of that nature is unnecessary. Do you view this approach as being basically different from an approach to healing that does involve touching?**

No. I believe they are similar, if their underlying purpose is to awaken within people a fuller awareness of the Spirit of God deep within them. This is what Jesus did. His way was to help people feel and sense their closeness with God, and he used touch, spoken commands, forgiveness, and compassion to do this. As I understand it, the Science of Mind approach to healing is primarily affirmative prayer, the purpose of which is to help people become aware of their unity with God.

I do believe, though, that physical touch can be a sacrament, that is, it can effect a sense of contact with the power of God. As I said before, Jesus used this approach extremely effectively. On the other hand, I recognize that the same "message" touch conveys can be communication through thought or through the mind. For example, once when my wife was in a severe accident and nearly lost her foot, I used a method of placing my hands around—but not touching—the injury. This followed our taking the sacrament of Eucharist together, symbolic to us of our union with God. I prayed that my feeble, natural healing power be multiplied infinitely by the divine healing power and would bring about the changes needed in order for her to be well. She would feel pain in her foot where she could usually feel nothing. She now walks without a limp.

For people who are active in denominations or in individual churches that do not have a healing tradition, what advice would you give them for developing such a program?

First of all, they might read my book *Psychology, Medicine and Christian Healing*. Then they will be prepared to view spiritual healing as a genuine Christian practice and will understand the value and legitimacy of it. With this background established, I think the next thing for them to do is to start reading the New Testament. They need particularly to read the four Gospels and to see how many instances of healing are described there. Forty-one different stories of healing are contained in the New Testament.

132   Then I think people interested in starting a healing ministry in their church need to look for somebody to talk to and pray with on this subject, so they don't feel alone. For the minister who wants to start a healing ministry, it would be good to have a person who is already experienced in carrying out a healing ministry come to the church. There is, for example, the Order of St. Luke's, which is an interdenominational order devoted to healing and which can provide good speakers to awaken the congregation.

What would the church do then?

The next step is to develop a prayer group. I think that a church without a prayer group is like a human being without a heart. A prayer group is saying that God is real—that God is still active in the world and that the Holy Spirit can change people in ways that enhance their lives. This is one of the great things that the Science of Mind has done. It has shown us that we can relate to the divine, that we are instruments of the divine, that we are aspects of the divine. The prayer groups should consist of people of a common mind gathered together to recognize God's presence. They will naturally begin to pray for the sick. A healing service can then be instituted, not as a main service of the church, but rather at a special prayer group time. For the sacramental churches, I'd like to have the Eucharist, the Holy Communion, to say that God is within our midst and sharing Himself with us. Following the Communion service, people could come up for the laying on of hands. Over the years, I have seen what amazing things can come from this practice.

And if the individual church really is opposed to this ministry?

In my opinion, a church cannot take Jesus' ministry and teachings seriously and not have a healing ministry. After you have shown people this fact, you can begin the ministry in a very quiet way. The minister doesn't have to come in and tell a person, "I'm going to lay hands on you." The power of the Spirit will work anyway, so you just need to pray. And where there are people in the congregation opposed to the idea of having a healing ministry in the church, it's important that you not make it the main service. For example, don't institute the healing ministry during the eleven o'clock service on Sunday! Have it at another time.

What can each of us do personally to develop our inner heal- *133*
ing potentials?

We need to write down what we really believe about the world. Do we believe that this is purely a materialistic world? Because if it is, and that is our basic belief, nothing we do in the healing ministry would be anything but nonsense, superstition, or compulsive action. The tragedy is that most Westerners don't believe in the spiritual dimension. Secondly, once one really believes in that dimension, he or she must find the nature of the Divine. My own deepest experience here is that God is love and that Jesus gave up Divinity, became a human being along with us, and suffered our pain and eventual Crucifixion. He showed us that this can all be transformed in the Resurrection. If this isn't love, I've never heard of love. That plus the story of the Prodigal Son are stories of the nature of God.

Next we need to have our own prayer life, in which we keep in touch with that Love. I think it is nearly impossible to be a significant spiritual healer unless one keeps in touch with and is an instrument of divine Love.

Is there any other advice you would like to add?

We have to live in love toward others to be consonant with the divine Lover whom we are supposedly serving. I also think we have to see life going on beyond the grave and realize the utter fulfillment of God's healing is in the hereafter, not just on this earth. A worldview that ends with the grave can give no real, ultimate healing to body and mind. Finally, if we are going to have a real healing ministry, we have to have the courage to take risks.

9 RELIGION AND SPIRITUAL HEALING IN AMERICA TODAY

AN INTERVIEW WITH J. GORDON MELTON, PH.D.

BIOGRAPHY

J. Gordon Melton is an ordained minister in the United Methodist Church. He took his master of divinity in Church History from Garret Evangelical Theological Seminary in 1968 and his Ph.D. in the history and literature of religion from Northwestern University in Chicago in 1975. Dr. Melton is currently the director of the Institute for the Study of American Religion and serves on the faculty of the University of California at Santa Barbara, where he is a visiting scholar in the Department of Religious Studies. An acknowledged expert both on the history of American religion and small religious groups, he is the author of the three-volume and authoritive *Encyclopedia of American Religions* as well as several other books. These include *The Dictionary of Religious Bodies in the United States; Why Cults Succeed When Churches Fail; The Cult Experience: Responding to the New Religious Pluralism* and the *Encyclopedic Handbook of Cults in America.*

J Gordon Melton is not the type of religious figure with whom the general public is too familiar. He isn't a TV evangelist and doesn't write popular books on using religion for better living. Dr. Melton is a scholar and historian of religion in the United States, with a personal library on the subject unequaled anywhere in the world. I first met Gordon in Chicago several years ago, when he was the book review editor for *Fate* magazine, on whose editorial staff I also served. But why interview a scholar on religion in a book on healing? The rise of New Thought philosophy in the nineteenth century brought spiritual healing back into religion more forcefully than ever before. It is the spiritual grandfather of "positive thinking" movements of every kind. So I thought that some background in the history and the future of religious healing should be included in this book.

For some time now, Gordon has been working out of the University of California at Santa Barbara, a pleasant drive up the coast from my home in Los Angeles. But finding Gordon posed somewhat of a problem. Like most scholars, he likes to immerse himself in his books — currently housed at the U.C.S.B. library, where he has his desk. I felt like a mouse in a maze, weaving my way through the book stacks to find him. But with all the difficulty, the setting — highlighted by the musty order of books of bygone years — was perfect for the interview.

D. SCOTT ROGO: Religion in the United States seems to go through cycles. Church attendance was at its highest in the 1950s during the Eisenhower years. Then we had the "consciousness explosion" in the 1960s and church attendance fell off, while interest in Oriental religions came to the forefront of popular culture. Just where are we now in the ongoing cycle of change?

J. GORDON MELTON: I tend to think we're dealing with long-term trends rather than cycles. The long-term trend is that Christianity is

136 continuing to grow and that church attendance has leveled off. I believe that growth of Oriental religion in this country was due primarily to a legal change in 1965 that, for the first time, allowed Asians to immigrate. The so-called "consciousness explosion" emerged from the large number of Asian teachers who came here after 1965.

It must be remembered that this country didn't become fifty percent Christian until the 1940s. Christianity in terms of church membership had always been a minority religion in the United States. It just had very little competition and what little competition it did have at the beginning of the century was suppressed by the Oriental Exclusion Acts—a series of laws instituted between 1917 and 1924 which cut off Oriental immigration altogether. So Christianity had its own field in which to grow and it had a protracted time in which to do it.

Are they any *specific* trends in American religion that you find notable?

The growth and public presence of Fundamentalist and Charismatic religions is quite obvious. The percentage of such denominations is not growing but their overall following is. What's important is that they are becoming publicly noticeable through the use of television. That is certainly a significant trend. On the other hand, the large liberal religions are continuing to lose members and are becoming somewhat spiritual dry holes. I think it's going to become very, very difficult for them to recover. The other trend I see is the growth of alternative religions of various kinds which — in the long term — are going to become major competitors to the Christian dominance.

That reminds me of a poll taken by the *Daily News* in Los Angeles a couple of years ago. It showed that the middle class overwhelmingly considered itself religious and maintained spiritual values, but didn't feel any need to be linked with a formal religion. So I'm wondering: Would you consider that we Americans — as a whole — are a particularly religious people?

I think we have become one. At the time of the American Revolution, for example, we were a tremendously secular people, a nonreligious people. We had a lot of legislation regarding individual rights and separation of church and state during those early years because of this wide-scale secularization. What we've seen happen in

America is that it has gradually become more church-oriented, more religious, and more outwardly observant of religious values and religious goals. So yes, I would say Americans are overwhelmingly religious. Most of them are church members, and the spread of religion is a very important part of American life. On the other hand, it is interesting that the two prime spots where religion is *not* popular happen to be two very powerful centers, namely, the campus and the newspaper office. Media people, reporters, and professors — as a whole — are the most irreligious people in American society.

You were saying that the large, liberal denominations are declining, while more fundamentalist or experiential ones seem to be becoming popular or at least more visible. Do you think some forms of organized religion are simply not meeting the spiritual needs, or the deeply personal needs, of the general public?

That's the major problem with liberal Protestantism. It isn't meeting the religious needs of its members, and therefore, large numbers are leaving and going to other churches. But a large number of lay men are hanging in there because they are fourth-generation Methodists or fourth-generation Baptists, for example. These people *are* finding ways to meet their needs without leaving the church.

Do you think the American people are inherently religious?

Yes, I do. People in general are inherently religious. Among the signs I can cite are the large number of experiences that we would call psychic or paranormal — for example, encounters with preternatural beings, surviving remnants or spirits of people they had known in this life in the body. For a hundred years we have been taking polls among various kinds of people about ostensible encounters with the dead, experiences of clairvoyance and telepathy, and other psychic and spiritual experiences. These are the kinds of incidents out of which religion is often made.

People have these kinds of experiences in large numbers. The recent poll by Father Andrew Greeley, published in the January/February 1987 *American Health* magazine, indicates that such experiences are just as common today as they were when similar polls were first taken. There's every reason to believe that people are really having these experiences and that they've become a normal part of their lives. Forty-two percent of Father Greeley's participants,

138 for example, claimed to have experienced spontaneous contact with the dead, while twenty percent reported visions. These data are consistent with a 1985 Gallup poll that showed forty-five percent of the public report deeply personal, religious experiences. Because of the overlay of secularity in our culture, most people don't talk about such experiences to everybody they meet, but these experiences become the basis for their personal spirituality. If these people find their way into a formal church, they and their experiences become integrated into a religious doctrine. If not, they just hold to their experiences, which give a spiritual overlay to their lives.

One phenomenon I find to be a uniquely American pattern is that this country perennially gives rise to so many religious movements, denominations, cults — short-lived and long-lived. Are there any religious or cultural reasons why we seem to initiate so many religious movements?

Religious freedom, and we are really not all that unique in this respect. Every place in the world where there is any degree of religious freedom the same phenomenon occurs. For example, hundreds of different groups are rising in Japan, thousands of different groups in India, and over five thousand groups in Africa south of the Sahara. Another factor is the rise of urbanization, since these movements are overwhelmingly urban groups. The only place you can find them is in the cities, so everywhere you have an urban mass you have religious groups forming. Many of them will be local to that particular city. So freedom of religion and urbanization are the two main factors that promote the rise of new religious groups.

Some of these "new religions" end up being called cults, some of them are called sects, some get labeled denominations and others are simply referred to as religious movements. Are there unique distinctions as to which religions receive which labels?

There very much are. I'm currently teaching a course on what I call "Cults and Anti-Cultism in America" at the University of California, Santa Barbara, and one of the problems we've had to deal with is what constitutes a "cult." We took a week discussing that one problem because there are so many definitions.

The term "cult" is primarily a negative label that other people stick on a religion. About half of the religious groups in America have been called cults at one time or another by different people. *139* Technically a cult is a group that has a religious life and structure quite distinct from that which is dominant in the culture. Thus in India you have the passing of anti-cult laws which are directed against such groups as Presbyterians, Methodists, and Catholics! In this country, Indian religions are often considered cults, and people likewise attack Maharishi Mahesh Yogi, Rajneesh, and the like. Sects, however, are generally considered intensely conservative forms of the dominant faith. Thus, the Evangelical Methodists are considered a sectarian group that came out of what became the United Methodist Church. The Orthodox Presbyterian is a very conservative body that emerged from the Presbyterian Church.

These various terms — sect, cult, and so forth — all have different meanings, but I've personally found them not to be helpful in the long run in doing my own work in teaching American religion. It's much more helpful to describe these groups in terms of the world's religious traditions, and I see various groups as representing those religious traditions in America. And, importantly, even though most of the major American traditions have been present throughout this century, many have only become widely visible as national organizations since 1965.

Why do some of these originally small movements succeed, while others fail completely?

For much the same reason businesses do. There's a very competitive religious marketplace in this country. Most of the new religious groups that come along are poorly organized and tend to be led by shallow teachers. Many of them deal primarily with the concerns of late adolescence and early adulthood and have no ability to adapt to the middle-aged or to the many things one has to confront if the movement tries to become a second- or third-generation religion, i.e., the education of children or even the presence of children within such an intense group. Just as many businesses die because they are undercapitalized, religious groups die because they don't have a place to build a full religious life as they grow. It is also very difficult to grow if the group is completely at odds with the dominant religious culture. So the more a group can fit in with the dominant religious culture of the land, the easier it is for them to succeed.

There was an incredible cultural milieu in the late nineteenth century that gave rise to several religious movements that

140 **became highly successful. The three that immediately come to mind are the Mormons, Adventism, and the whole rather populist religious ideology that became known as New Thought.**

Right.

So I'd like to discuss New Thought and how it evolved. First of all, can you define what the New Thought movement is?

New Thought began in the 1880s. It was basically an attempt to deal with a number of intellectual problems present at the time as well as a number of practical problems—such as the poor state that medicine had fallen into and never gotten itself out of. We were still in a circumstance where it was probably healthier not to go to a doctor than to go to one! But New Thought was also an attempt to build an alternative worldview, primarily one that was positive. It was based on what was called a monistic world vision—that is, the view that everything, the basic reality of the world, is spirit. It served as an alternative to what was then called materialism, the idea that the basic "stuff" of the world was material, and that whatever we think of as nonmaterial was a lesser "fluff" thrown off from the material world.

This monistic view of the world—in the West, anyway—began with Mary Baker Eddy and it grew out of her successes and out of the work of her students—many of whom later left her. Her students often attempted to soften the absolute position she took about the reality of spirit and the unreality of matter, trying to find a more moderate approach to that issue. Basically, however, they agreed with her that spirit was the essential reality and that matter was a lesser reality, and many of them did go all the way with her in saying that matter was unreal.

But one of her students in particular, Emma Curtis Hopkins, took a lot of ideas that had originated with Eddy's students, those who had left, and pulled them together into a movement, which became what we know today as New Thought.

So until that time, New Thought was really a very loose-knit cultural movement more than anything else?

Yes. New Thought was actually a name that was coined in the 1890s. Until that time its proponents were still calling it Christian Science. For example, when Charles Fillmore of the Unity School of Christianity came along after playing the religious field, he decided these were correct teachings. He originally called his journal *141* *Christian Science Thought* and only later changed it to *Unity.*

At that point in the 1880s, before Hopkins came along, there were a number of people laying out ideas that came together to make New Thought—Emanuel Swedenborg, the Swedish mystic of the eighteenth century, was probably the most important progenitor, followed by Phineas P. Quimby, Warren Felt Evans, who is often cited, and many others. Even the world of popular Spiritualism contributed to it, and while New Thought people rejected the belief in contact with discarnate spirits, the idea that spirit was the dominant reality certainly came into New Thought teachings. But Emma Curtis Hopkins was the person who pulled it together. She became the great teacher and among her students were the founders of all the great New Thought schools and, of course, her last student in the 1920s was Ernest Holmes, who developed the Science of Mind philosophy.

There were actually two main influences on Ernest Holmes, one was Emma Hopkins and the other was Thomas Troward. How do you regard their respective contributions to Ernest Holmes's philosophy?

While New Thought had developed in the 1880s and 1890s, we must remember that it was only in the late 1890s that the idea of the subconscious mind, which is so important and integral to our thinking today, was presented to the American public by William James and later by Sigmund Freud.

Thomas Troward was an Englishman who had been a judge in India, and when he retired he returned to England and brought with him some Oriental teachings. But at the same time he was reading such writers as William James, Thomson J. Hudson—the author of several books on hypnosis, the subconscious, and psychic phenomena—and the French psychologists who were developing the idea of the subconscious. What Troward did was to revise New Thought philosophy into a form which included the recognition of the subconscious. New Thought writings prior to that time included no concept of the subconscious. But Troward did include it, and that was the great contribution he made to New Thought.

Ernest Holmes immediately recognized the value of Troward's work and integrated it into his own ideas. Holmes, after absorbing New Thought from a number of teachers, began to teach Troward's philosophy soon after he encountered it, around World War I. Then in

142 the early 1920s, Holmes encountered Emma Curtis Hopkins. The major contributions Hopkins seems to have made to Holmes's thought were in terms of her mysticism. When you read Troward's writings, you find cold analysis, while one encounters in Hopkins a warm personal side which she seems to have passed on to Holmes. In Holmes's writings we find this combination of the cold scientific analysis characteristic of Troward as well as the personal mystic side.

Do you think the New Thought philosophy as such is still a viable force in American religion today?

It has had a very vital presence since the turn of the century, and it still does. For example, over half of the religious bestsellers in this country have been New Thought-style books. In the 1930s, it found its way into the mainstream through people such as Glenn Clark, Norman Vincent Peale, and in our own day, Robert Schuller. Norman Vincent Peale's contemporary, Louis Dunnington—who was a Methodist— popularized it and then it was intertwined into the Jewish community through people such as Joshua Lichtenstein. So apart from its roots within New Thought groups and its development into organized churches such as the United Church of Religious Science, Religious Science International, Unity, Divine Science, Home of Truth, and a host of independent centers, it also was adopted as a religious philosophy within more traditional systems of belief. This philosophy has, in general, found a vast audience in the present day.

What do you regard as the most important contribution of New Thought teaching?

I think the great contribution New Thought has made—and of course I include the Science of Mind philosophy here, as well—is its ability to empower people who feel, for whatever reason, that they are powerless. New Thought has shown an amazing ability to speak to these people and teach them about their inner resources, to teach them what their own negative approaches and vision of the world is doing to them. By getting a more positive outlook on life, these people are developing a greater sense of their own worth and a greater sense of their own capabilities. They are empowered to make use of their inner talents and to turn sickness into health.

What about the relatively affluent middle class? What is the main message such a perspective particularly offers to them?

It tells the upwardly mobile that their striving is correct. It points out to them that this is not a dog-eat-dog world, but a spiritual universe. They recognize that if they ignore their moral principles, if their upward striving is at the cost of their honesty and it harms others, then ultimately they themselves will be done in. Their striving will have been for nothing.

Two other areas come to mind where the New Thought viewpoint can be of help to people. One is in providing a viable alternative to orthodox religious teachings, when those teachings have proved to be too confining or limiting. And another is in pointing out a way by which a person can have direct spiritual experience, without the need for go-betweens or formal religious structures. Can you comment on those?

Certainly such religions provide an alternative to mainline Christian orthodox thought. However, we must remember that "orthodox" has two meanings—one, the traditional teachings of the church and the other, the mode in which those teachings are held. Any set of teachings, be they Christian, Buddhist, or even the Science of Mind, can be held in such a way that they become limiting instead of freeing.

On the second point, I tend to think that direct spiritual experience, unmediated by "go-betweens or formal religious structures" is almost nonexistent. Now, what do I mean by that? Most of us have significant, extraordinary, mystic experiences. But without the availability of other people who have had similar experiences and who can assist us, we have no way to explain them—to integrate them into a world of meaning.

What future do you as a religious historian see for the New Thought teachings in our culture?

The Science of Mind teaching, as a religious philosophy, comes as close as anything I know to being in tune with the American character, with what we generally call "the American way of life." It will be with us for the rest of our lifetimes, certainly as long as this country is heading in the way it is currently going. What kind of organizational forms it may take is very difficult to predict. But there will certainly be a New Thought movement and there will probably also be an increasing number of people who imbibe this in order to put it to use in their lives.

10 CAN PSYCHIC HEALING BE LEARNED?

A VISIT WITH LARISSA VILENSKAYA

"There is enormous interest there!" Larissa smiled as she spoke. The brownhaired and affable engineer was relatively new to the United States and seemed a bit nostalgic for her former homeland.

I was talking about parapsychology and healing research in the Soviet Union with Larissa Vilenskaya, who was formerly one of the Soviet Union's top researchers. Our meeting took place at the Washington Research Center, which was then a privately endowed parapsychology laboratory near downtown San Francisco where Ms. Vilenskaya was working. She had emigrated from the Soviet Union in 1979 so that she wouldn't have to cooperate with Soviet officials, who wanted to conduct unethical types of psi research, i.e., research on telepathic mind control. Leaving the Soviet Union guaranteed her freedom in her choice of research.

When I learned in 1981 that Ms. Vilenskaya was working in California, I couldn't resist the opportunity of flying to San Francisco from my home in Los Angeles. My goal was to learn about recent Soviet parapsychology and healing research from one of the best-informed spokespersons available in the United States. There were several subjects I wanted to explore, but I left Los Angeles with few expectations about what I would eventually learn. Nor did I know much of Ms. Vilenskaya's background except for an interview with her that Henry Gris and William Dick, two American journalists, had published in their book *The New Soviet Psychic Discoveries*. (I was to learn from Larissa that the interview was a fabrication and that she had never met with the authors.) Far from the ponderous, regimental,

and ivory-tower scientist I expected to find, Larissa—as she asked   *145*
me to call her—turned out to be friendly, relaxed, lighthearted, and
insisted that our talk be informal. I was so interested in her information about Soviet parapsychology that I returned to San Francisco a
month later to formally interview her.

Larissa was born in 1948 in Riga and at the age of nineteen began
her formal scientific training at the Moscow Steel and Alloys
Institute, Department of Semiconductor Materials and Devices. She
studied there until 1972 and specialized in electronics. From 1967 to
1975 she also worked at the A. S. Popov Scientific and Technological
Society for Radio Engineering in Moscow, where she was affiliated
with the Laboratory for Bioinformation (a Soviet term for ESP), and
where she eventually directed the lab's Experimental and Training
Group. During 1975–76 she worked as a research assistant at the
Institute for General and Pedogogical Psychology, Academy of
Pedagogical Science of the Union of Soviet Socialist Republics in
Moscow before emigrating to Israel for two years. While an Israeli cit-
izen, she entered the United States in the summer of 1981 on a
tourist visa in order to attend the Second World Congress on Science
and Religion, which was scheduled in St. Petersburg, Florida. She
had been in correspondence with Henry Dakin (the same Dakin of
stuffed toy fame), who funded the Washington Research Center. He
was interested in having Larissa working there, which provided her
with the impetus to move to the United States permanently.

Larissa first became interested in parapsychology and psychic
healing when she was still a student at the Popov Society. In 1967
she had the opportunity to witness an exhibition by Karl Nikolaiev
and Uri Kamensky, a well-known telepathic "team," who have been
working with Soviet scientists for several years. They had come to the
Society to lecture on parapsychology and to give a demonstration of
their abilities.

"The test was made in two different rooms," Larissa reminisced.
"It was a kind of telepathy test under not very strict conditions.
Kamensky was given an object to send to Nikolaiev telepathically. It
was some sort of metal chain or necklace. But a friend of mine had an
interesting idea. Maybe we could interfere with the session and send
our *own* image. It was our idea to do this to prove whether this was all
some sort of stage performance or magic trick, or whether we were
really seeing the interaction of human minds."

146   The two students decided to concentrate on sending Nikolaiev, who was isolated in a separate room, the image of a magnet. They concentrated for several minutes on a magnet Larissa had borrowed from the physics department. They had, of course, no way of knowing what the telepath was reporting from his station in the other room. The results of their little experiment were only known when the demonstration had been concluded.

"Everything Nikolaiev said in the other room was transcribed," Larissa continued. "Afterwards we found out that he first began by describing the necklace—long, metal, golden color—but then began to describe our magnet as rectangular, metal, grey, and gave its approximate shape and so on. Then later, as he finished the session, he came back to the magnet. This proved to us, two people with no experience, that we could interfere with a telepathy experiment and make a successful transmission."

This first exposure to psychic phenomena sparked Larissa's interest and she began systematically studying parapsychology. Her first opportunity to experiment with a gifted subject came some time later when Rosa Kuleshova, who specialized in fingertip vision, visited the Laboratory for Bioinformation. Larissa worked extensively with Kuleshova, whose remarkable powers later became worldwide news. The young engineer was able to document Kuleshova's talent for identifying colors with her fingers even when the samples were placed under several layers of transparent paper and she was blindfolded. When she told Larissa that she had *learned* this ability while working with the blind, the engineer became even more excited. She began toying with the possibility that she could develop similar powers as well.

"I tried," she explained, "and though I can't say I learned to read with my fingers, I was successful at identifying colors, large letters, and so on."

Larissa was soon training other subjects in this peculiar skill. Most of them were young women employed by the Laboratory. While they eventually learned some degree of skin vision, Larissa's interests soon turned to psychic healing.

"In 1969," she explained, "I met a psychic healer who was also working at the Laboratory for Bioinformation. He said that I could do healing myself, and that he could see whether people had this ability. I was a young girl, about twenty, and couldn't even think about it at the time. I later began my first attempts at dermal vision, but we *147* eventually discovered that the development of dermal vision led to a sensitivity of the hand in general to the human biological field—the aura—and the capability to make diagnoses. Dermal vision was a direct route to psychic healing."

Larissa began working with several people who had successfully learned skin vision and learned that several of them could feel a slight "prickly" feeling when they placed their hands near, but not touching, the human body. She felt that this sensation was produced by an interaction between her subjects' hands and the human biofield. On the basis of this discovery, the young investigator began training her subjects to diagnose and heal by interacting with this field.

"We learned," Larissa went on, "that a person with no complaints has a biofield which is more or less regular. But if the patient had some disorder, even if the person making the diagnosis didn't know about it, the healer still felt a distortion of the biofield. He could not explain it in medical terms, since we were working with people with little medical knowledge. But they would be able to note where the patients had problems, inflamations, or previous operations."

Larissa began experimenting herself and found out that she, too, could diagnose and heal. On one occasion, she explained, she was working with a woman who suffered from reticulitis. Her pain was so bad that she had been bedridden for two days. While running her hands near the patient's body, Larissa was stunned to find practically no biofield whatsoever connected to the woman's throat. She made a mental note of the disturbance but said nothing to the patient. She instead treated the woman's pain by sending healing energy to her. The treatment was so successful that the woman was able to leave her sickbed. Larissa then cautiously inquired whether the woman suffered from a throat problem. The patient was stunned, for she suffered from a lifelong thyroid disorder which was being controlled by medication.

"This kind of experiential attempt taught me that it was really possible to do this sort of thing," Larissa added with a grin.

I was particularly interested in psychic healing since such research has been at the forefront of Soviet psi research. Unorthodox medicine *in general* is popular in that country, since Soviet medical technology is not exactly the best. The Soviet Union is literally filled

148 with psychic healers. Larissa's former Moscow roommate, Barbara Ivanova, has publicly lectured on her healing powers and has demonstrated her talent for making psychic diagnoses before several eminent Soviet scientists. Then there's Juna Davitashvili, who has regularly treated up to one hundred patients a day in Tbilisi, and has become a present-day folk heroine. Another famous resident of the city is Alexey Krivorotov, who—with his two sons—has been so successful with his healing work that a medical conference was held in Moscow in 1976 to discuss research with the family. Lesser known in this country is Vladimir Safanov, who can purportedly diagnose a person from his photograph.

What is so surprising is that this work is not kept secret like much Soviet psi research, but is common knowledge. Healing research in the Soviet Union has none of the cloak-and-dagger elements that in the past have typified Soviet parapsychology.

"Is there any reason why, of all areas of parapsychology, this one is being pursued in depth?" I asked.

Larissa responded immediately. "In Russia medical care is free, but on the other hand, it isn't on a sufficiently high level. So people try to seek relief in nontraditional ways including psychic healing. And there are also several people around who can successfully demonstrate it."

She continued by explaining that two levels of interest in healing research exist in the Soviet Union today. There is, of course, public interest in finding and making personal use of psychic healers. But there is also *official* interest in healing since even some top-ranking Soviet officials have relied on psychic practitioners when necessary. Soviet government officials have, in return, sanctioned publication of favorable articles on psychic healing in the popular press. These reports, which have even included interviews with the healers themselves, have encouraged both public and scientific interest in the subject.

Larissa kept emphasizing throughout our talk that popular interest in psychic phenomena and healing is enormous in the Soviet Union, even though information isn't easy to find. In fact, a few years ago Larissa surveyed the Soviet public on their interest in psychic phenomena by asking the respondents if they possessed psychic powers. She found that 43 people of the 122 polled believed that they possessed such capabilities, with telepathy and healing the most commonly claimed psychic powers. A good percentage of these people felt that psychic talents could be learned, but even more of them felt that they were inherited.

I knew of this wide-spread interest in psychic phenomena in the Soviet Union, but when I asked Larissa why she felt popular interest was so rife, I was surprised by the response.

"Religion is forbidden in Russia,"* she explained. "There is no way to express or satisfy the desire to know more about ourselves, the world, and other levels of perception. No one takes materialistic philosophy seriously. It's the funniest thing. Everybody studies courses in materialistic philosophy and passes exams on it. This is obligatory in high schools and universities, but *no one* takes it seriously. People want to understand what is beyond all this, what understanding we can have of the world, of human nature, and of the universe in general."

I was intrigued by what Larissa was saying since I had long wondered whether Soviet scientists or the general public was interested in the evidence for life after death. This is an aspect of parapsychological research that is looked upon with disfavor in the Iron Curtain countries. Back in 1973 I was engaged in research on out-of-body experiences with the Psychical Research Foundation in Durham, North Carolina, under the laboratory's director, W. G. Roll. Roll had recently returned from a conference in Czechoslovakia, where he had presented a report on survival research. The paper and every reference to it were later censored from the conference's published proceedings. My meeting with Larissa served as an opportunity to explore underground survival research in the Soviet Union.

Larissa explained that little information on phenomena such as hauntings and poltergeists is publicly available, but that some scientists were beginning to take an unofficial interest in survival phenomena. These researchers have been playing with procedures similar to table-tilting and Ouija boards.

Reincarnation research is one of the few phases of survival research that has received some public promotion, due in part to some aspects of Larissa's own experiments.

"It was not an official study," she began by commenting. "It was work by Barbara Ivanova and myself along with some friends and colleagues to satisfy our interest. We made some regressions and tape-

---

* This has begun to change with *glasnost* — D.S.R.

150 recorded the sessions. We tried to find some, not verification, but pertinent observations. For example, one of our subjects saw himself living in a place where people spoke Czech, German, and Hungarian in the last century. He is a physicist and in this life he had studied both Czech and Hungarian... which are totally useless for his work. One young girl in a reincarnation session described herself as a rich woman in a rich apartment but in a strange dress. She described the dress. She held her hands above her legs and spoke about how strange it was that her hands didn't lie on her legs."

The subject was not well educated and didn't know that women of that period wore dresses that ballooned out—just as she described.

"Of course, it was difficult to rule out subliminal memory," Larissa warned me, "but it was interesting to us as indirect evidence for reincarnation."

Even more fascinating was the public's response to Larissa's published research.

"We managed to publish small parts of our work in the local newspapers along with translations from the Western press on reincarnation in a very abridged form," Larissa explained. "We learned later that these clippings had been cut out and passed from person to person."

Interest was so widespread that the young researcher was soon being asked to lecture on her experiments in several Russian cities.

"There were people who were skeptical," she told me, "and people who were interested. But there were very few who didn't care or who were indifferent."

Of course, lecturing on something as bizarre as reincarnation was not easy in the Soviet Union, where anything smacking of religion or metaphysics was then condemned. Even telepathy could *only* be publicly discussed in terms of "physical waves" or information transmission. It could not be couched in terms of thought transmission or any other metaphysical models. So while Larissa was able to publicly present her findings, she could only proceed by skirting the metaphysical issues they suggested. She presented her research by calling them interesting experiments in the *acquisition of information* concerning previous lifetimes rather than in terms of the soul's rebirth.

Nor was it long before the Soviet scientific establishment came up with a purely materialistic explanation for Larissa's data. One physicist suggested that the individual biofield probably contains information coding that person's life. This field may only slowly disintegrate upon his or her death. Another individual could possibly connect to that field years later and pick up information regarding past places, eras, and people.

Larissa also explained that reports of phenomena such as ghosts and hauntings are barely known in the Soviet Union. A poltergeist report was run in a Ukrainian newspaper in the 1920s, but the general feeling in the Soviet Union is that such outbreaks result from spontaneous psychokinesis, or the power of mind over matter. Everyone in that country is familiar with Nina Kulagina, the Russian housewife who can move objects simply by concentrating on them, and stories about her powers have been widely published in the Soviet press. Since the existence of such powers has become commonly accepted in the Soviet Union, any sort of spiritistic or demonic explanation for poltergeists is simply unknown... or at least never discussed.

Larissa left the Soviet Union in 1979, with hopes that she could conduct parapsychological research without state interference. She worked first in San Francisco translating Russian scientific manuals, but she has not yet returned to her first love. She still hopes to return to parapsychology. Before I left the Washington Research Center, I asked her what research projects she would pursue if given the chance.

"I would most like to work with psychic healing," she answered. "I would like to objectively determine the existence of the healing ability. When we worked with people in Russia we didn't exclude the possibility that our subjects were responding to psychotherapeutic effects. We didn't know what part of the effect was psychological and what part was psychic healing. We tried to help people and that was all. I participated in a few short studies with people suffering from hypertension, though our subjects didn't know I was trying to help them. I was on the other side of the room sitting with some papers. I didn't do anything visible, but just tried to influence them. Blood pressure readings were taken before and after the sessions. In most patients, it was lower afterwards. So I'm interested in finding some biological detector—some system in the body—that would be sensitive to human psychic influence... to see to what extent it is possible to develop healing abilities."

Today, Larissa lives in Monterey, where she works as a teacher and

152 Russian translator. Her interest in parapsychology and healing have never diminished and she edits *Psi Research*, a scientific periodical on parapsychology, published by the Washington Research Center.

PART III. | WAYS TO HOLISTIC HEALTH

11 | THE HEALING REALITY

AN INTERVIEW WITH DEEPAK CHOPRA, M.D.

Dr. Deepak Chopra took his original medical training in India before coming to the United States, where he received additional training at hospitals connected with Harvard, Boston University, and Tufts University. Board certified in internal medicine and endocrinology, he was formerly chief of staff at New England Memorial Hospital in Stoneham, Massachusetts. He has also served on the faculties of both Boston University and Tufts. His interest in Eastern healing traditions led him to study Ayurvedic practices, a form of holistic medicine stressing meditation, sound therapy, and herbal supplements. It also led him to become the founding president of the American Association for Ayurvedic Medicine. As well as lecturing internationally on his work, Dr. Chopra has written such books as *Creating Health: Beyond Prevention, Toward Perfection, Return of the Rishi: A Doctor's Search for the Ultimate Healer,* and *Quantum Healing: Exploring the Frontiers of Mind-Body Medicine.* His latest book is *Unconditional Life: Mastering the Forces that Shape Personal Reality.*

The drive from Los Angeles to Santa Barbara is particularly pleasant since it passes many miles of undeveloped coastline and rugged hills. It was a perfect way to prepare for an interview exploring the nature of reality. Dr. Chopra is an Indian-trained physician who has given up conventional medicine to reinstitute the traditional healing practices of his native land. The story of his journey through medicine is told in his wonderful book *The Return of the Rishi* (wise man). This was followed by a more speculative book, *Quantum Healing*, which serves as the basis for this interview. Dr. Chopra was staying in a picturesque and regal Spanish-style hotel right on the beach, and he cut an incongruous picture with his informal dress and ethnic features. He apologized for being a little late for his interview. His seminar had run overtime, he explained, and we had to rush to the airport. Talking together in a coffee shop there, we were occasionally interrupted by overhead jets and an incessantly running electric blender. Maybe it wasn't the best setting for the interview, but in typical meditative style, Dr. Chopra transcended the distractions with perfect mindfulness.

D. SCOTT ROGO: Could you explain to our readers a bit about your cultural background and your medical credentials?

DEEPAK CHOPRA: I took my medical degree in New Delhi. I then came to the United States and received training in internal medicine and endocrinology and metabolism at hospitals associated with Harvard, Boston University, and Tufts. I was eventually board certified in internal medicine and subsequently in endocrinology and metabolism. I am a fellow of the American College of Physicians and I've taught on the faculties of Boston University and Tufts. I've been in private practice the last twelve to fifteen years.

As for my cultural background: I grew up in India, where I was

exposed to a lot of Ayurvedic [traditional Indian] healing traditions.
However, I did not pay any attention to them until I got involved in
meditation, specifically TM™. I subsequently went back to India in
order to rediscover my own traditions.

**What led you, after your medical training, to take an interest
in meditation?**

I had a busy practice. I was making lots of money. I would come
home in the evening, ask myself what did I do? Did I make a difference in anybody's life? I had spent my whole day writing out prescriptions mostly for antibiotics, antihypertensives, tranquilizers,
sleeping pills, drugs for treating ulcers, etc. I knew I was not doing
anything for the patient, merely masking the symptoms of illness
while the underlying process raged on, many times worse than before.
I tried something else. I started telling my patients, "You've got to
stop smoking, stop drinking so much, lose weight, don't be so
stressed, don't get so angry, so impatient, learn to laugh, stop being so
serious." They would say, "My mother-in-law says the same thing.
She doesn't charge me fifty dollars to tell me this stuff. Tell me how to
do it."

We know all the right things. We know what's good for you, what's
bad for you. It's the how-to that's missing. We have great outer technologies, no inner technologies. I began to search. In my own culture
and tradition I discovered that seers and sages had perfected techniques over thousands of years. These were techniques of awareness.
The rishis of India were masters of inner awareness. They had developed exquisite subjective knowledge, and along with it exquisite
control, of both mind and body. Meditation was the key to inner
awareness. I was having my own problems experiencing stress and
burn-out. I decided to try meditation.

**What sorts of experiences did you have in meditation that
led you to question the Western medical ethic?**

The Western medical ethic is based on the knowledge of parts. Its
very methodology reinforces isolation, separation, fragmentation. I
did not have any sudden insights or "satori" experiences in meditation but a gradual evolution of my own understanding of the scheme
of nature. It was an experiential knowing of which I had not the
slightest doubt and its basic tenets could be summed up as follows:

158   Our physiology is the physiology of nature. We sing because the universe sings, we create music because the universe is music, we dance because there is a cosmic dance, we dream because the universe dreams, we make images because the universe creates through imagination. We breathe, eat, digest, metabolize, eliminate, because this is an alive, breathing, eating, digesting, metabolizing, eliminating universe. Our intestines are the bowels of the earth, our gonads the earth's self-replicating machinery, our eyes and ears its antennae, and our thoughts quantum events of the unified field. We are gloriously entrained, intertwined, inextricably bound to, interconnected, part of, the intricate patterns of the whole universe. We cannot separate ourselves from this web of life. When we struggle to do so—we feel unwell—sick. Sickness, disease is a self-correcting signal to realign the patterns that structure the whole. Separation, alienation, isolation, fragmentation are not part of the natural scheme. The part contains the whole, the whole is encoded, embedded in the parts— any deviation from this pattern automatically self-corrects. The symptoms of this self-correcting procedure may be experienced as discomfort, disease, unhappiness, etc.

These insights seem almost grand when expressed verbally. In a sense they are not at all intellectual concepts but simply a nonverbal knowing in the quantum mechanical body-mind, a quiet exultation that this is the way things are and all we have to do is go with the flow. It is a silent "Amen," a joyful "So be it."

From reading your writings, it seems to me that you are trying to interface Western allopathic medicine with what some people call "spiritual" psychology. For example, recently you wrote that "the doctor must make an inner journey, taking his understanding beyond the limits of the physical body and into the heart of a deeper reality." Could you elaborate on this provocative remark?

In the Western model of reality, our entire reality is structured out of our perceptions. Now according to my own cultural tradition, that is only one *type* of reality. From a purely scientific perspective, too, it is becoming obvious that what you and I experience as perceptual reality is, in fact, merely a small segment of what's out there. This concept has even been demonstrated in the psychology laboratory. You can raise a group of kittens in a room with only vertical stripes and they grow up seeing only a vertical world. This phenomenon has nothing to do with their belief systems. Within their brains, the internal neural connections permit them to see only vertical or horizontal stimuli. In other words, the sensory exposure that we have when we are growing up permits us to interpret our universe in a certain way. There's even a technical term for this phenomenon: *premature cognitive commitment.* The fact remains, however, that the universe is not material in its essential nature. What you and I call matter is a response of the observer, a function of our perceptual apparatus. This perceptual apparatus freezes the universe into what we can call the "objects" of perception.

The concepts you are espousing seem consistent with some concepts used in subatomic physics.

The world is made up of atoms, which are particles moving at lightning speed around huge empty spaces. These particles aren't material objects, but fluctuating fields of energy in some universal field of energy. But as long as we are stuck in our perceptual mode, we can only see that limited worldview. The eye of the honeybee only sees honey at a distance because its eye cells are not sensitive to the usual range of colors. A snake senses its environment through infrared radiation. A bat senses its whole universe through sonar. What's the real picture of the world? There isn't such a thing. In order to go beyond this perceptual artifact called "reality," we have to make an inner journey. That can only come by transcending the senses, by entering that field of awareness where, experientially, we recognize that mind and body are essentially manifestations of one field.

Based on that expanded structure of reality, I take it that you feel traditional Western medicine is extremely limited in its outlook?

Yes. Traditional Western allopathic medicine is based on what you might call the "frozen sculpture" model of the world. It's a materialistic concept based on Newtonian physics—in other words, we are outsiders and perceive the world from this independent perspective. We are not seen as insiders or part of nature. Based on this materialistic framework, Western medicine has developed "magic bullets" to treat diseases. If you can't believe you "ate the whole thing," have a couple of Alka Seltzers. If you are suffering from a headache, take an

160 aspirin. If you can't go to sleep, take a sleeping pill. If you are feeling anxious, take a tranquilizer. If you are experiencing chest pain, take a nitroglycerine tablet. For cancer we have chemotherapy. For infections we have antibiotics. We have "magic bullets" for instant gratification to release us from our symptoms without really ever getting to the source of disease.

Probably the form of healing that you most emphasize in your writings is Ayurvedic healing. Will you explain the philosophical basis of these practices?

The entire notion behind Ayurvedic treatment is different from the Western concept that we are machines that think. It teaches that it's the other way around: We are thoughts that have learned how to create the physical machine, the body. We are fluctuations in consciousness that manifest in the form of matter. We are part of the universe. There's a very nice expression in Ayurveda that basically summarizes this conceptual framework. It says, "as is the atom, so is the universe / as is the microcosm, so is the macrocosm / as is the human body, so is the cosmic body / as is the human mind, so is the cosmic mind." And healing occurs spontaneously when the human mind entrains with the Cosmic Mind. So what we call mind and matter are essentially the same thing.

Do you feel that this model is scientifically justifiable?

From modern science we are learning that this model is, in fact, true. On a quantum level, your body is made up of atoms. This is a river of atoms, not a frozen sculpture. The Greek philosopher Heraclitus said that you can't step into the same river twice, because new water is always flowing by. That is true of the body. You cannot "step" into the same flesh and bones twice because new atoms are coming and going. The human body is a dynamic field of energy that is constantly in exchange with the rest of the world through several processes: eating, breathing, digestion, metabolism, and elimination. But most importantly are our thought processes: feelings, emotions, desires, instincts, drives, ideas, and concepts. These processes structure your reality of the body right at a molecular level.

Let me try to make this clearer. To make a thought is to make a molecule. To think is to practice brain chemistry. It is now recognized that the biological equivalents of our thought processes are the neuropeptides in the brain. But these neuropeptides are not just in the brain but pervade every cell of the body. They are our immunomodulators—chemicals that regulate the body's immune system—as well. To make it even more complicated, it now turns out that the cells of the body are, in turn, capable of making the same chemical messengers that the brain produces when you think. So when you have a gut feeling about something, you are no longer speaking metaphorically but scientifically. In other words, your gut is making the same chemicals that your brain would make if it were having the same reaction. So mind is no longer confined to the brain, but literally pervades every cell of the body.

What are the medical or related practices used in Ayurvedic treatment?

The practices used in Ayurveda to evoke the healing response rely on our internal pharmacy—the body's capacity to make immunomodulators, anticarcinogenic drugs, antihypertensive drugs, and any other drugs you could think of. The stategies we use are the following:

First is meditation, which lets you settle down to a silent state of awareness, beyond thought, to the experiential level of total unity with the universe. You experience the fact that you are part of the larger wholeness. Remember that "thought" is what separates us from each other and from the rest of the universe.

Second is psychophysiology. The patient learns at that silent level of awareness to introduce specific impulses of intelligence into the body to evoke physical responses.

Third is primodial sound, which is a way of using sound so that consciousness can transform it into physiological responses from the body.

Also used in Ayurveda is sensory modulation. According to this tradition, we are the end product of our sensory experiences... which come by way of sound, touch, taste, and the other senses. So we modulate these sensory experiences to specfically elicit the healing response. Utilized in this respect, as I mentioned earlier, is sound therapy and aroma therapy. We also use special massage procedures called *marma,* which focus on specific points on the body that influence functions elsewhere. These are known as junction points of consciousness and matter. It is also interesting that the Ayurveda recognizes six tastes—sweet, sour, salty, astringent, bitter, and pungent—

162 which influence our physiological responses. So we use food as medicine. In other words, we use everything that happens to us as experiences to evoke different kinds of healing responses.

Is there anything else specific to Ayurveda?

There are other techniques which use herbal supplements to enhance the immune system or evoke other types of physiological responses—such as slowing the heart rate, changing blood pressure, and so forth. These herbal supplements—which we are currently studying from a scientific framework—stimulate ongoing processes in the body. They don't add anything from the outside. In Ayurvedic terms, they stimulate the intelligence of the body, which is the ultimate and supreme genius mirroring the wisdom of the universe. We also have procedures for removing toxins from the body, since on a material level, they represent the metabolic end products of our experiences and stress.

When we combine these approaches, there are roughly twenty of them, we have a system that deals with the body in every aspect.

As a physician trained in Western medicine, what results have you seen with a treatment so inconsistent with Western concepts of healing or "cures"?

Let me cite the more dramatic results and then the less frequent ones. The most dramatic results we see consistently are the following: Eighty percent of people who come to the doctor's office complain of headaches, stomach aches, insomnia, or anxiety. These are know popularly as psychosomatic illnesses. With these conditions we have excellent results right across the board. But let's talk about other diseases which aren't generally felt by Western medicine to be *that* influenced by psychosomatic factors—such as heart disease, hypertension, bronchial asthma, or rheumatoid arthritis. We find extraordinarily good results with all these illnesses using Ayurvedic techniques. Recently we have even seen some very dramatic spontaneous remissions in cancer. We just wish it was more consistent! We feel it will be when we understand the exact mechanism behind such results. Recently, we've introduced Ayurvedic concepts to our clinics in San Francisco and New York for the treatment of AIDS. We're getting very good results in terms of patient comfort and the frequency of opportunistic infections, to which these patients are prone.

It is obvious that you feel that mind influences the body even *163* **more dramatically than is commonly recognized in modern medicine.**

Not only that. I believe that at a quantum mechanical level, the mind and the body are essentially the same thing. I feel that mind and matter are essentially two sides of the same coin—which is consciousness.

There is a point of confusion here, however, that I'd like to clear up. If you say that the mind influences the body, some people might think you're saying that the brain controls the healing process. That could imply that the brain is the mind, which is a completely materialistic concept.

The brain, in my way of thinking, is the transducer of a universal field of energy. It really doesn't matter *what* you call it, but the universe consists of a creative field of energy. Now according to physics, the forces of nature can be classified into four primary categories— the strong and weak nuclear forces, gravitation, and electromagnetism. In some way these forces resolve into a unified field. We believe that this unified field is a field of intelligence and that the "mind" is not confined to the brain, nor even to the body. It pervades the entire cosmos. Our brains merely structure our thought processes, which represent limited aspects of a more universal mind.

Do you have any idea by what mechanism the mind controls the body via the brain?

Yes. I think the mind manifests itself as the neuropeptides, which are the raw materials for what structures brain activities. I would make an analogy here to a computer. Your body is the printout. Your central nervous system is the hardware. The biochemistry of the nervous system, the neuropeptides, is the software. Your mind—your feelings, thoughts, emotions, and so forth—is the programming. But then there's the programmer. And that programmer is this field of consciousness, your inner self. It is consciousness that first conceives, structures, governs, and then becomes the body's physical matter—including the brain cells.

I'd like to turn now specifically to your book *Quantum Healing: Exploring the Frontiers of Mind-Body Medicine.*

164   **One of the principal themes of the book, from my reading, is that a person's reality system contributes to disease. Can you elaborate on that notion?**

Our reality is structured through a process of social and cultural indoctrination, which one scientist has referred to as the "hypnosis" of social conditioning. In other words, our interpretations literally *become* the molecules of the body. For example, you can take a group of mice and give them an immunostimulant and have them sniff camphor. After a while, the mice will smell camphor and stimulate their immune systems. It's similar to a Pavlovian response. Similarly, you can take another group of mice and give them a drug that destroys the immune system and then have them smell camphor. In the future, the mice will destroy their immune systems when they smell camphor. Now is it the camphor that is destroying or stimulating the immune system? No. It is the result of the way the mind and body interprets the stimulus, the smell. That interpretation literally determines the physical reality of the body and ultimately the person's perception of the world. That obviously relates to disease processes, too.

What exactly is quantum healing?

The word *quantum* means the smallest indivisible unit in which waves are emitted or absorbed. This is the definition of Stephen Hawking. For example, a quantum of electricity is an electron. A quantum of gravitation is the so-called graviton. A quantum of light is a photon. A quantum of mind is thought... an impulse of intelligence. What I call quantum healing is using one mode of consciousness, the mind, to bring about changes in another mode of consciousness, that is the body. It brings with it a sense of unity within the body. Another concept I like to use is that it brings about peace instead of violence in the body.

Could you cite an example of quantum healing from your own practice?

I could cite many examples. The most dramatic was a recent case. The patient had breast cancer with metastasis to the bone. It pervaded her skeleton, skull, everywhere. Yet today she is free of cancer. Her blood chemistry, which indicated earlier that the cancer had spread to the liver, is normal. Her CT scans are normal. Her skeletal survey is normal. In other words, she does not have cancer.

How did this cure come about?

She employed all the techniques we talked about earlier.

If the mind is so inherently linked to the physical body, does this imply that it is linked on some level to the universe in general?

Yes. As I've tried to emphasize, I think the mind and the body are two aspects of the same thing. What we experience as matter is only an artifact of our sensory experience. As long as we tie our reality to sensory experience, we're stuck with a limited reality. The universe is a field of infinite possibilities, infinite transformations, and our bodies are part of it. The body is not really static, but a river of intelligence. Biologically, you make a new skeleton every three months, a new liver every six weeks, a new skin once a month. So if you think you are your physical body, then you really have a serious problem! The 1989 model is completely different from the 1988 one.

As we come to the close of this interview, let me ask you what I feel to be an important question. Even with its many problems, Western medicine and technology have done a pretty good job of keeping people alive. Maybe we can't cure some diseases and conditions, but we can manage them. Why, then, do you think it is important for people to explore alternative forms of healing... whether it be Ayurvedic or any other system?

First let me respond to the first part of your statement. We like to give Western medicine credit for keeping people healthy, prolonging their lives, and improving the basic quality of life. But the most significant advances in the prevention of disease and for better living have occurred because of basic measures unrelated to medicine. These would include better sanitation, better nutrition and, to a small extent, vaccination. These are the reasons we enjoy better living today. Not antibiotics, not chemotherapy, not drugs. So I would give Western medicine a little less credit than you.

I do not, however, discard Western medicine completely. But if I look very carefully at the data I'm confronted with, I recognize that ninety percent of all prescriptions used in today's medicine—four billion prescriptions written yearly—are for "optional" or marginal use. That means they don't make a bit of difference to the natural his-

166 tory of a disease. Secondly, if you look at last year's statistics collected by the Rand Corporation, you find that 100 billion of the 500 billion dollars spent for medical treatment was wasted on useless high-cost technology. But I still would maintain that there are situations where you can and should resort to drugs.

And in response to the second part of my question?

I think we have to look at the whole universe that exists inside us, the quantum mechanical universe. When we really begin to understand it well, we won't be requiring these interventions that introduce violence into the body.

Is there a single issue that has primarily guided your work, your books and seminars?

Let's change our interpretation of the material universe, as well as our interpretation of the material body. When we change this interpretation to better conform to a quantum mechanical framework, we'll receive the insight that this body is not merely made of molecules. It consists of transformations of energy within a universal field of energy. Once we recognize this fact, we'll find our bodies to be much more dynamic, exciting, and controllable."

12 | HEALING YOUR LIFE THROUGH SELF-ACCEPTANCE

AN INTERVIEW WITH LOUISE L. HAY, D.D.

BIOGRAPHY

Louise L. Hay, D.D., is best known today as a metaphysical teacher, counselor, and writer. She completed her ministerial training with the Church of Religious Science in New York and took a Doctor of Divinity degree from Science of Mind College. She subsequently became a Science of Mind practitioner there. In 1976 she wrote a unique booklet entitled *Heal Your Body*, which listed more than 150 mental causes for physical illnesses and offered metaphysical ways of overcoming them. The booklet received international acclaim and was translated into nine languages. Ms. Hay settled in southern California in 1980, where she wrote her book *You Can Heal Your Life*, which was later listed on *The New York Times Book Review* best-seller list for three months. Her most recent work has been helping people with AIDS and her latest book is entitled *The AIDS Book: Creating a Positive Approach*. She has also prepared several tapes of her teachings and exercises, which are distributed (like her books) through Hay House in Santa Monica, California.

I had long wanted to meet Louise L. Hay, since she is nearly a folk hero in Los Angeles. When the AIDS epidemic "officially" struck in 1981, there was virtually nothing, medically, that could be done to help people with the disease. Louise Hay was one of the few who stood up and said that there *was* something the sufferers could do. By giving empowerment to these people, she initiated a "fight back" attitude that has come to typify many people with AIDS. This wasn't a completely novel suggestion, since Dr. Hay is a Science of Mind practitioner, which emphasizes positive thinking. But the sheer power of her personality and message made her a cult figure in the AIDS community and offered PWAs (people with AIDS) something conventional medicine (then) could not: hope.

Since Dr. Hay's background is old-fashioned New Thought metaphysics, her office in Santa Monica seemed incongruous when I first visited it. It is modern and chic and serves as offices both for her organization and her publishing company. Dr. Hay struck me as a more mature person than her pictures in the press indicate, but she still displays the beauty that made her a successful model in New York. Because she writes so many books for the general public, some people have criticized her for being "superficial." But as I spoke with her, it was clear that she has a well-grounded background in metaphysical philosophy and has taken on the role of popularizer deliberately and, I might add, very successfully.

D. SCOTT ROGO: What personal experiences originally led you to take an interest in the Science of Mind philosophy and the United Church of Religious Science?

LOUISE HAY: I originally heard about Science of Mind from a friend and decided to check it out. The first meeting I went to was in New

York City at the Church of Religious Science on Forty-eighth Street. Raymond Charles Barker was the minister there, though he wasn't the one who spoke that day. What I heard really intrigued me. People told me that if I was willing to change my thinking, I could change my life. It was the first time anyone had ever told me that. The first-year classes were taught on Wednesday afternoons and Thursday nights and I took both trainings. I kept going and going and going because it interested me intensely.

How did that experience lead you to become a Science of Mind practitioner?

I was so fascinated that I continued to study everything I could get my hands on. The next thing I knew, three years had passed and I was eligible to apply to become a practitioner. I took the tests and passed. Almost immediately I had a full-time practice.

I understand from your book *You Can Heal Your Life* that your involvement with the Science of Mind helped you to overcome cancer.

It certainly gave me the tools to work with; when I had the problem I realized what I needed to do, what I needed to clear, and I reached out for help.

Tell us the story behind your self-healing. How did you first discover that you had cancer?

I had a vaginal problem that was not healing properly, so I consulted with some doctors and they did a biopsy. When the results came back there was evidence of a malignancy. They wanted to operate immediately but I bargained for time. Knowing surgery was only one possible solution, I wanted to see what else could be done about the situation. I consulted with a very good nutritionist, who helped me detoxify my body, and I did a lot of work with Eric Pace, who was my teacher at the time in New York City. He was invaluable to me. He was out here in Los Angeles when I was first diagnosed and I called him saying, "Eric, they tell me I have cancer." He said, "Louise, I don't believe you have accomplished all the work you've done just to die from cancer. This is a challenge for you, something for you to overcome." When he returned to New York, we did a great deal of

170 work together. I also went to a therapist, though not a conventional psychotherapist, and worked to clear out a lot of old garbage I had been carrying for a long time from my childhood, when I was badly abused.

All these approaches combined to enable me to overcome the cancer within six months.

You have become well-known for your books and tapes that help people cope with illness and disease and improve their lives. How would you summarize the essentials of what you teach?

There is one Presence and Power in the universe that is with us at all times and which we can use for our benefit. What we give to life is returned to us, and what we believe about ourselves becomes our reality. Those are some central points in my philosophy. Above all else, though, I like to emphasize that we are all worth loving.

What other beliefs are important in your philosophy?

I list several of these beliefs in the first chapter of my book *You Can Heal Your Life*. For example, I believe that the universe totally supports us in every thought we choose to think and that the Universal Power never judges or criticizes us. I also believe that our personal power is always operating in the present moment and that the way we exercise this personal power is through our thought. By changing our thoughts we can change what we experience.

Most of us have negative or limited ideas about who we are and as a result we limit the good that can come into our life. We focus on thoughts that include resentment, criticism, guilt, and fear instead of thoughts that help us to feel loved and valued. But we can change that, and when we do, our life improves.

You teach that a lack of self-love is a central cause of the unhappiness many people feel with regard to their jobs, relationships, and lives in general. What do you think contributes to this lack of self-love?

I think it comes from not believing that we really deserve good and therefore not aligning ourselves with the Power for good in the universe, with God. We discount ourselves. And if we engage too much in this type of thinking we aren't going to attract positive experiences. *171* I find that when people are willing to work on loving themselves, they begin to attract good things. In my own life leaning to love myself has brought tremendous changes for the better.

Are there specific factors that lead people to resist self-love?

Yes, there are. And often these factors are the result of our early childhood environment. Many people never knew love when they were children since they were constantly criticized or put down or abused by their parents. They were viewed as being inadequate in some way. Being good little children, they simply accepted that verdict, even though it wasn't true. It was just someone's opinion.

Is there anything that can be done to correct those early feelings of not being good enough?

One way those feelings can be changed is through being willing to forgive. I find that people who have difficulty loving themselves usually need to do some forgiving. If it is hard to love yourself, usually there is someone in your life who's done something to you but whom you haven't forgiven—and maybe that person is yourself.

Are there exercises you could recommend for learning self-love?

The essential and most important step is to stop criticizing yourself, now and forever more. Self-criticism doesn't do any good and it breaks down your inner spirit. Begin to accept yourself exactly how you really are and make it OK to be whoever you are. Stop feeling negative about your sex, age, weight, the job you have, or the relationship you're involved in. Start right now to love who you are and accept yourself. Out of that experience, positive change can come into your life.

Earlier you mentioned the importance of learning to forgive. Could you elaborate on the role of forgiveness in self-healing?

I think a lot of people sit in what I call a prison of self-righteous resentment. Somebody did them wrong and because of that, either they want to get even or they refuse to forgive the person. But they

172 themselves are the ones locked in prison. To forgive somebody doesn't mean to condone his or her behavior. It simply means to set yourself free.

We have to give up any resentment we feel, and this process has nothing to do with other people. They may not even know we're forgiving them. But when we're willing to let go—when we forgive—a whole weight drops from us.

We've been discussing the need for self-love and forgiveness and the role they play in our life. How does the lack of self-love and forgiveness relate to the onset of disease or illness?

The cells of the body react to the emotional environment in which they live, just as you yourself do. For example, if you went to an office every day and your boss screamed at you and said everything you did was wrong, you would be under terrible pressure. Let's say, too, that it was a filthy office. I can guarantee that you would not do your best work. There's no way you could. But if you went to an office where you were loved, respected, and appreciated, and you could blossom at what you did best, then wonderful things would happen in your work.

The same process works inside the body. If the cells in the body—which are doing their best to keep you healthy—are living in an atmosphere of continual criticism, fear, anger, and resentment, they are eventually going to become sick. It would be very difficult for them to maintain health in that sort of environment.

Are there different approaches you would use to help a person overcome a medical problem rather than a purely emotional or life-related one?

Not really. I learned a long time ago that when I focus on helping people love themselves, the changes for the better were so dramatic that I stopped the other approaches. I use mirrors with people a lot. I find that mirror work is extraordinarily powerful. If you look into the mirror and say "I love you" and all sorts of terrible feelings come up or you get angry or start to cry, you become very aware of how alienated from yourself you have become.

The universe is always here to provide us with good things in life. But when we don't feel good about ourselves, we in effect put up blocks that keep us from experiencing those good things. We don't let that wonderful flow happen between us and the universe.

I observe in your book *You Can Heal Your Life* that positive
affirmations play an important part in your work.

Yes. Positive affirmations to me are like short spiritual mind treatments. They are both the same sort of thing, in that they help us become aligned with the spiritual truth about us—that we are inherently divine and therefore whole and perfect.

What we need to remember is that every thought we think and every word we speak is acted upon by the Law of Mind. Far too many of those thoughts and words are very negative. If we can begin thinking and speaking in an affirmative manner—making positive statements about everything and every aspect of our life—our experience has to change for the better.

Could you give us some examples of general positive affirmations that people can readily use to improve their lives?

Well, I can give you a few I use.

That's certainly good enough!

One I frequently use is: "I know that everything I need to know is revealed to me." This affirmation takes a lot of struggle out of my life. If I am supposed to know something, then I will know it! And I'll know it when I need to know it. I don't have to read every word of every newspaper, since any information I require will come to me at the appropriate time.

Another affirmation I use is: "Everything I need comes to me in the perfect time/space sequence." In saying this to myself, I know I'm always being supplied by life with whatever I need.

A few more are: "I am safe wherever I go," "I am loved," "I know that I am constantly prospering." I also like this affirmation: "My income is constantly increasing." I've used that one for years and it has been very good to me.

Others which are very effective are: "I have wonderful relationships wherever I go," "My body is constantly healthy." And finally a good general affirmation is to say: "All is well in my world."

Now I'd like to put you on a benign sort of hot seat for the moment. I'd like to bring up some possible criticisms of these approaches to solving problems and see how you respond to them.

174   That's fine.

To begin with, by saying that people cause their own illnesses and other problems in living through their negative thinking, aren't you laying a "guilt trip" on them?

The entire basis of the Science of Mind is that we create our own reality, but the point of this teaching is not to make people feel guilty when something undesirable happens to them. Rather, the point is to help people understand that they have the power to change their experience.

If we can use the power of our thought to create negative experiences, such as disease, unsatisfying jobs, or inharmonious relationships, we can use it to create a fulfilling, joyous life for ourselves. My goal is to lead people toward greater freedom, not burden them with a sense of guilt. As I said earlier, we always need to be willing to forgive ourselves for thoughts and actions that perhaps weren't wise and to realize that we were doing the very best we could at the time.

I find that people who choose to be guilty regarding a particular situation in their life are usually people who tend to feel guilty about everything. Now they are giving themselves another reason to feel guilty. The ideas I teach do not involve laying blame on anybody but rather they help people deal with negative circumstances in a responsible way... to make use of the inner power we all have, through our unity with God, and resolve the problem.

The approaches we've been discussing focus primarily on improving the self. I'm wondering how a person avoids becoming "spiritually narcissistic" while relying on these techniques. By concentrating on his or her own life and growth, isn't there a danger that a person will lose concern for other people or society's problems in general?

I don't see that happening at all. To me, people who truly love themselves will neither hurt themselves nor other people. I find that when people can really improve their lives on an inner, spiritual level, they want to help other people. They become more socially conscious. It's when we are frightened, angry, and isolated behind walls that we are not interested in other people. But if we love ourselves, then we are much more open to loving others.

One of the things I want to accomplish is to help create a world where it is safe for us to love one another. It's very important to me to live in a world where we can love and accept each other exactly as we *175* are. Then we can relax and simply be the best that we can be. If it's OK for you to be who you are, you are going to relax and become more of you. But if I start criticizing you and pointing out where you're wrong, you are going to clam up on me. I think we all do that in our lives.

The work in which you are currently involved and for which you have been widely acknowledged has been with people with AIDS [PWAs]. What first led you to become interested in the specific problems faced by PWAs?

Well, it just happened. In my work as a practitioner of the Science of Mind, I had a few clients who were gay, and occasionally somebody would call me and say something like, "Louise, I have a friend who has AIDS. What do I tell him?" I soon realized that if I were simply to tell the caller the main points of my philosophy, much of the importance might be lost when that information was imparted down the road. Something might be lost in the translation. So I decided to make a tape called *AIDS: A Positive Approach.* One side of the tape consisted of my ideas at the time on how we contribute to disease and the other side included exercises for deep relaxation and guided meditation. That tape very slowly began making the rounds. Remember that in the early days of the epidemic, I was the first person who said anything positive about AIDS. Everybody else was pointing to gloom and doom, but I didn't believe that everybody with this disease had to die—and I still don't believe it. Even in the days of the Black Plague not everybody died. Many people did, but not everybody.

Didn't this initial work lead you to form a small group of PWAs?

Yes, a few people came to me and asked me to start a small group. I started with six people in my living room and that was just over four years ago. I told them that I didn't know what we were going to do but that we weren't going to sit and play the game "Ain't it awful." We knew what the media, the government, and the medical profession were saying; however, we wanted to see what we could do from a positive angle. So we began to gather positive information. We also did a lot of work on releasing resentment, worked on forgiveness, and learned to love ourselves. We always ended the session with spiritual mind treatment.

176 **What was the result?**

After the first night, one of the participants called to say that he had enjoyed his first good night's sleep in several months. So that little group began to grow, and today we still meet every Wednesday night in West Hollywood and we have about eight hundred people there.

I was just about to discuss these meetings in West Hollywood with you. Your Wednesday night "Hayrides," as they are lovingly called, have become known throughout the world.

Yes, people have been coming from all over the world, because there is really nothing like them anywhere except for the New York branch I have. I have a very good teacher in New York who does a large group there. Remember, though, that it is not a healing meeting as much as a support group. We support people in being who they are, overcoming challenges, and improving the quality of their lives.

Would you describe a typical meeting?

There really isn't a typical meeting. They vary continually. We're beginning to have people who are homeless and who have AIDS coming to us, which is a challenge that is stretching us. We do a lot of sharing, with people expressing their fears and feelings. I talk for awhile and we bring up pertinent issues. We do some singing and meditation, and I always end the meeting with a prayer or spiritual treatment.

You mentioned previously that you're not striving for physical healing in your work. We know there's no cure for AIDS—

I don't agree with that statement. When you say there's no cure, you're merely pointing out that the medical profession, at the moment, hasn't come up with a chemical that will kill the virus and not kill the body. But I don't agree that there's no cure. There are some people who are getting well from AIDS. It is a limited number and we can't yet identify what specific thing they've done to overcome the disease. If we found that out, obviously we could have everyone do it.

Let me rephrase the question I was going to ask. Since there

is no immediate cure for the disease, what are you primarily
hoping to accomplish in your work with PWAs?

I'm helping people to go through a time of intense crisis and terror
in the most comfortable way they can. We provide support for them. I
know a cure for this disease will be discovered, even though we
haven't found it yet.

So you feel we will eventually overcome AIDS?

Everything is eventually overcome! Look back into history.
Nothing lasts forever. I think the breakthrough could happen much
sooner, though, if people would take a more positive attitude about
the possibility of conquering AIDS.

**What gives you the inner resources to carry on with your
work, writing, and practice?**

I'm deeply grateful to the Science of Mind background I've had
and have. This background has given me a rock to stand on in times
of intense crisis. Even though the earth may be shaking all around
me, I have inner knowingness that is very strong for me. The Science
of Mind has given me a feeling of safety and connection with the universe. I feel very safe in life. I'm deeply grateful for the training I
received, for it has given me the opportunity to do the work that I'm
now accomplishing on a scale I probably couldn't have done otherwise. That's something I often think about.

When you look at my background and early childhood where I was
so abused, and see where I am now, it shows the tremendous changes
that can take place when people love and find themselves... when
they learn to use the principles that govern the way life works. That's
the most wonderful thing that Ernest Holmes did. He gave us the
opportunity to understand just how life works and I love it. I love
being able to help people.

13 THE POTENTIALS OF THERAPEUTIC TOUCH

AN INTERVIEW WITH JANET F. QUINN, PH.D., R.N.

B I O G R A P H Y

Janet F. Quinn, Ph.D., R.N., is an associate professor of nursing at the University of South Carolina. Dr. Quinn has been involved in the practice, teaching, and research of therapeutic touch since 1976. She has given therapeutic touch workshops throughout the United States and in Canada; been a guest on radio and television programs in the United States, Canada, and England; authored numerous articles and book chapters; and received the first federal research grant to study the effects of therapeutic touch. Her current research is exploring the impact of therapeutic touch on the immune systems of both recipients and practitioners.

Everybody knows the soothing effect of human touch. Whether it is a formal massage or a gentle squeeze on the shoulder, touch is an important form of nonverbal communication. But is there more to touching than purely this psychological dimension? Therapeutic touch is the practice of psychological and physical healing through either direct contact or merely by bringing the fingers near to another person. Research into the physiological parameters of the effect is now over a decade old, but research into the healing power of touch received an important impetus in 1979 when Dr. Janet Quinn—a professor of nursing at the University of South Carolina—published her first important research on therapeutic touch in the *American Journal of Nursing*.

My chance to interview her came when we were both invited to talk at a parapsychology conference in Atlanta. Janet was extremely tired after a day of travel and lecturing but gladly granted the interview. She explained that it was time to *stop* talking to the scientific community and "get the word out" on the power of therapeutic touch to the public. That evening, we snuck out from the party our hosts were throwing and conducted this interview, hoping we wouldn't be missed.

D. SCOTT ROGO: What exactly is therapeutic touch?

JANET QUINN: There are probably lots of ways I could answer that question, but the easiest is to see it as a derivative form of laying on of hands, since the procedure uses the hands with the intent to heal. Therapeutic touch was originally developed by Dolores Krieger and Donna Kunz. Dr. Krieger is a professor of nursing at New York University and Dora Kunz has for many years been a healer in her own right. Dr. Krieger developed this system by watching the very well-known Canadian healer, Oscar Estebany, and then trying to imitate him, by following the directions given by Kunz. She wanted to

180 see if she could learn how to do healing. It turned out that she *was* able to do it.

Exactly what procedure does a person use when performing therapeutic touch?

Dr. Krieger has identified certain steps one goes through. First there is what's called *centering*, which basically entails shifting your consciousness from the everyday world to a more internal, quiet perspective. Some people call it a meditative state. From there, one moves into an *assessment* of the patient. This evaluation doesn't simply mean looking at the person's physical, psychological, or emotional state, since we make an assumption while working with therapeutic touch that people represent fields of energy. So the assessment focuses on perceiving the way this energy is flowing and is distributed in the patient. This is done by moving the hands over the patient's body. Following this assessment procedure, there is an attempt to *rebalance* those areas of the person's energy field that don't appear to be "balanced," by either touching them directly or moving the hands over them.

So therapeutic touch involves working with some kind of energy.

Apparently. However, I want to emphasize that the idea that we're dealing with an energy is really only a working hypothesis. While that's the model we're using now, it's important to know there's little scientific evidence to support that concept in any substantial way. So this energy model must remain hypothetical until we can demonstrate it scientifically. Clinically and experimentally, however, people performing therapeutic touch experience it very much as though it involves an energy. They feel some sort of energy moving through them and can feel it around other people. So the hypothesis is meaningful for us.

What kinds of research have been done into the effects of therapeutic touch?

The original research in this area dealt directly with the laying on of hands and was designed by Dr. Bernard Grad, a biochemist at McGill University in Canada. Grad was able to demonstrate that the laying on of hands could increase the growth rate of plants. This

research was interesting since Grad conducted the experiment by *181*
having the healer treat water that was later used to irrigate the plants.
The healer wasn't anywhere near the plants themselves.

What other experiments did he conduct?

Dr. Grad also did studies with laboratory animals and demonstrated, in a really elegant way, that the laying on of hands increased their
rate of recovery. Mice were used for the experiment and small patch-
es of skin were removed from their backs. The mice treated by the
healer recovered more quickly than mice treated by other people who
didn't know how to use the laying on of hands and who merely placed
their hands around the cages.

Following this original work, there was more formal research on
therapeutic touch. Dr. Krieger worked with hemoglobin counts, and
she found that patients given therapeutic touch seemed to show
increased hemoglobin levels, which means their blood was oxygenat-
ed more thoroughly. Those studies, however, need to be replicated,
since they were early and rough. A later study, reported by Patrician
Heidt in *Nursing Research,* demonstrated that anxiety in hospital
patients was reduced through therapeutic touch. So that's some of the
background.

**Was there any other significant work before you conducted
your own research?**

There was the important work of Sister Justa Smith of Rosary Hill
College in New York, who worked with Oscar Estebany and the laying
on of hands. She showed that Estebany could influence the behavior
of enzymes in a sealed container.

**What are some of the more impressive physical effects
you've seen in people receiving this treatment?**

Before I answer that question, I want to emphasize that the focus
of therapeutic touch is the whole person. Our primary intent is not
necessarily to cure people of the signs and symptoms of their diseases. Rather, we want to help them move in the direction of wholeness and healing, which is likely to be more than merely eliminating
symptoms.

But the fact is—and I'm speaking clinically now, not from a
research perspective—we see certain physical changes. We see that

182 therapeutic touch really has an impact in terms of pain control. Many different types of pain respond very well clinically to therapeutic touch. I've personally had a lot of experience with people who have different forms of musculoskeletal problems—whiplash, injuries, arthritis, rheumatoid arthritis, and sprains. Therapeutic touch seems to accelerate the healing of those conditions very, very rapidly. Some of the side effects of chemotherapy, such as nausea, can also be effectively treated with the procedure. Tension and migraine headaches respond, and you could extend the list indefinitely. I can't list diseases that therapeutic touch cures because we can't make that claim. I can only report what, again speaking purely clinically, we seem capable of accomplishing with the procedure.

You said earlier that the energy transfer model, or energy manipulation model, is really only "axiomatic" to therapeutic touch. That is, it is assumed to be valid, but cannot actually be proved one way or the other. What alternate explanations can you give for the effects of therapeutic touch?

The most obvious is that we're seeing a form of self-healing, perhaps suggested by the healer's work. Now, some people might refer to this in terms of a placebo effect, a reference to the powerful self-healing mechanism we all possess. Maybe the person doing therapeutic touch somehow brings about this self-healing.

You seem to be suggesting that therapeutic touch can become a ritual by which a person releases his or her own healing ability for self-cure, but without taking responsibility for it.

Yes. In fact, I believe all healing is essentially self-healing. So if you take that as your first premise, then the rest of the problem involves trying to find ways to facilitate or bring forth a person's self-healing power. My goal is to find the way to release this power in the least invasive fashion, and I believe therapeutic touch is such a way.

Another way of explaining therapeutic touch is to see it in terms of a communication model—that is, the treatment is a form of ritual. But perhaps embedded in that ritual is a communication that tells our patients how we expect them to behave. The very movements of the hands become metaphorical in this regard. For example, if you have a

pain in a particular part of your body, I would begin to move my hand *183*
over it. My hand will look like it's pulling the pain right out of the
body. That's a powerful message to you to trigger your own self-healing. So you see, there certainly are ways to explain therapeutic touch
without relying upon the concept of some sort of energy transfer.

**From what you've said, then, is physical contact really nec-
essary for therapeutic touch to work?**

No, it's not. My own research was designed, in fact, to test that
exact hypothesis. If there's really some sort of energy exchange during the procedure, you shouldn't have to physically touch people. So
my research used therapeutic touch in which no physical contact
took place between the patient and the healer. The healers kept their
hands four to six inches from the person—yet we got the same results
as one gets using physical touch.

**It seems obvious, then, that therapeutic touch has both a
physical and a mental aspect to it. For instance, you talked
earlier about the concept of "centering." Can you describe
how you actually enter into this special state of consciousness?**

Centering is probably the most important part of the entire process, but it's also the most difficult to explain. When people are first
trying to learn how to do therapeutic touch, centering is quite difficult for them. It's really very simple, but most people have never
experienced such a state of consciousness before.

It's like telling someone, "Take a drive now and go see my friend
Sarah," but not saying where Sarah lives. That's all the direction you
give the person, who is left to drive around in hopes of somehow and
sometime arriving at Sarah's house. But if the person has been to that
place even once, getting back will be much easier. She'll at least
know where she's trying to go, even if she's not sure exactly what
route to take! Of course, it gets easier with repeated visits, when she
knows the direct route.

When people begin to learn to shift their consciousness into this
inwardly focused, calm—yet still alert—state of mind, they simply
have to learn the best way to find that space so they can return there
at will. We use exercises to help people learn to experience this state,
such as visualization procedures, guided imagery, and other tech-

184 niques. From there, it's a matter of the person's learning how to return until he simply "knows" how to be there.

Has scientific research verified the existence of this specific healing state of consciousness?

Research has indeed been done, though there are questions as to how the results should be interpreted. For example, a study was carried out at Langley-Porter Neuropsychiatric Institute in San Francisco by Dr. Joe Kamiya, who worked with Dolores Krieger. Dr. Krieger—as the person who was going to be performing the therapeutic touch—was attached with electrodes which led to an electroencephalogram. They also hooked up three patients to similar equipment and simply watched what happened.

During the therapeutic touch procedure, Dr. Krieger's EEG changed dramatically as soon as she began the healing intervention. It shifted into something called "rapid synchronous beta wave activity," which is a state of consciousness—or a brain wave pattern—which has been associated with Zen meditators. The patients with whom Krieger was working demonstrated a similar shift in their own EEGs within minutes of when Krieger began the treatment and began to produce a lot of high-amplitude alpha waves, even though their eyes remained open. That's unusual because we ordinarily associate that particular brain wave pattern with states of deep relaxation.

But even though that study has been done, the question still remains: Is Krieger's specific brain wave activity typical of the state? Is it exhibited by all practitioners of therapeutic touch? Or is it idiosyncratic only to Dr. Krieger? Those questions haven't been answered at the present time. Because of that study, some people refer to therapeutic touch as a form of healing meditation, but we simply don't know whether all healers enter into the same state of consciousness. Is the "centered" state only a single state of consciousness or does it comprise many states?

Also, the concept that therapeutic touch is contingent on a special state of consciousness is linked to the concept of *intentionality*, which seems to be pivotal to the procedure. Maybe it's not so much which state of consciousness a practitioner enters, but the *intention* of the practitioner while he or she is interacting with the patient. That's the real key. It may be that this centered state of consciousness we've been discussing allows the practitioner to focus *intention* to the patient, and that the shift in consciousness for its own sake is not what's really important.

If therapeutic touch actually does produce results, what are the implications in regard to such concepts as long-distance healing, so-called "absent healing"?

The fundamental idea behind therapeutic touch is that we don't stop at the boundaries of the skin. So, if we talk in terms of an energy exchange that occurs some four to six inches from the skin, we might also wonder if it occurs eight inches from the skin. Or ten inches. Perhaps it can occur across the room, the town, or the country. You have to ask: What are the limits of this influence? I don't think we know the answer to that question. But there certainly are people— Joyce Goodrich, for instance—who are doing research with long-distance healing.

In some forms of spiritual healing there is no physical contact, no energy exchange is involved, and distance is irrelevant. It is based on the idea that we are all rooted in a Cosmic Mind and what is known in one place in that Mind— an awareness of wellness, for example—can have an effect in any other place, whether across a room or across the country. Can you comment on that healing method in terms of your own research?

From your description, I do not see the two types of healing as necessarily incompatible. The fundamental ideas are, I believe, related. In fact, I think that at some point in the future we will realize that all of the "alternative" healing approaches are actually tapping into the same mechanisms but are simply using different frameworks and hypothetical constructions to articulate and explain them. For instance, we all acknowledge that there is more to health and to healing than our current biomedical model suggests and that there are approaches to healing which have barely begun to be understood although they have existed for centuries. The idea that we are all rooted in one Cosmic Mind, which some would call God, does not preclude an exchange or transfer of energy between the "thinker" and the "thought about."

As I continue to explore the ancient healing traditions across philosophies and across religions and across cultures, there are sev-

186　eral consistent principles which seem to emerge. One of these is the healing power, the healing capacity, of unconditional love. Whether we attribute this healing power of love to the great Cosmic Mind, to the All, to the Universe, to God, or to the individual Higher Self, the principle remains the same—love heals. So we return to the idea of intentionality again: What is the intention which I hold toward and for you as I lay my hands on or as I think about you across the country?

I'd now like to talk to you about your own research. How did you first get involved in therapeutic touch?

I needed an elective in graduate school, and therapeutic touch looked sort of interesting! That was when I was taking classes at New York University working toward my master's degree in nursing. Dolores Krieger was teaching it and I sat through the first half of the class with my arms folded across my chest. I thought it was the craziest, kookiest stuff I'd ever seen or heard. I was thinking that there was no way this could be real. But another part of myself just knew this was for me. It was difficult for me to feel that way because I was thinking this stuff was such nonsense.

I got through the semester, though, and in the process Dr. Krieger performed the procedure on me. It was then that I knew something very real was going on, so I continued to learn about it and practice it. I took more advanced workshops and started working on family members, patients, friends... anyone who would let me practice on them. And when I went back to school to get my Ph.D., I specifically wanted to do research on therapeutic touch.

What kind of research did you do then?

The study I did for my doctorate was on the effects of therapeutic touch on anxiety. It was a replication of an earlier study, but I didn't use physical contact between the healer and the patient. I reasoned that if therapeutic touch involved some sort of energy, rather than being based entirely on physical contact, you shouldn't really need to touch the patient at all.

So I went into a hospital and worked with a group of cardiovascular patients, who were divided into two groups. One group received real therapeutic touch treatment without contact. By "real treatment" I mean that the nurses who performed were centered and focusing on helping their patients. The other group of patients received a mimic form of the treatment. By "mimic treatment," I mean that the nurses used the same movements as the other practitioners, but they didn't really know how to implement therapeutic touch and they merely counted numbers—backwards from one hundred by sevens—to keep their focus on ordinary thinking. I measured the patients' anxiety levels before and after these interventions and found that there was a dramatic drop in anxiety for those who received the real procedure. There was no change in the group that received the mimic procedures.

How did you measure the anxiety?

There's a scale we use that measures state anxiety, and it is based on the patient's self-report. The scale consists of twenty statements such as "I feel calm," or "I feel jittery," to which the patients respond.

The most important thing about the research was that the treatments—real and mock—looked identical... I videotaped each of the nurses doing the real and the imitation touch and had them evaluated by independent judges. None of the judges could tell which nurse was performing which procedure. So here you have what *looks* like identical treatments, with the only difference being in what the nurses were thinking while working with their hands. That distinction alone was sufficient to account for the dramatic difference we saw between the two groups.

So therapeutic touch doesn't rely solely on a set of movements or a methodology; it's the specific intent behind the procedure that determines whether healing occurs.

I understand that after your research was reported, you received a government grant to study therapeutic touch.

I received a grant from the National Institutes of Health, Center for Nursing Research, to further study the effects of therapeutic touch on anxiety. This research was meant to be an extension and replication of the work I just described. I changed several aspects of the experiment, however. For example, I turned the patients on their sides so the practitioner was standing behind them. There wasn't any eye or facial contact between them, since I wanted to see if that kind of contact was necessary for therapeutic touch to work.

188   We're still evaluating the data, so I don't have any results yet, but this gives you an idea of the ways I'm going with this research.

Have you done any other research projects on the effects of therapeutic touch?

I recently finished another experiment, which hasn't been analyzed yet either, but it's a very exciting study funded by the Institute of Noetic Sciences in California. It's a study of the psychophysiological correlates to therapeutic touch—this time hands-on healing — displayed by both the patients and the practitioners. What we're looking for is the effect of therapeutic touch on immune system functioning and several psychological factors. My reasoning behind the study is that we're finding, from the field of psychoneuroimmunology, that positive emotions might strengthen the immune system. We already know that negative emotions could suppress it. So I wanted to see what happened to the immune system in people who frequently and consistently engage in acts of unconditional love and compassion—which is what therapeutic touch represents. For our pilot study, we used subjects who were recently bereaved because we know from the literature that their immune systems tend to be somewhat suppressed. Two very experienced therapeutic touch practitioners treated the subjects over the course of seven days. We did some measurements both before and after the treatment, and we'll be looking at what results are forthcoming.

I can see already, however, that there are very clear differences in the psychological data. But we're still in the preliminary stages of evaluating this study.

Do you see any spiritual implications in therapeutic touch?

When we talk about healing, we talk—as I stated earlier—about wholeness. When we talk about this wholeness, we have to talk about spirit. We have to talk about body, mind, and spirit. So when we're working with something like therapeutic touch, the whole person of the practitioner—body, mind, and spirit—is interacting with the whole person of the patient. Therapeutic touch is, in fact, *experienced* as being very spiritual. When you try to get into the business of "birthing" wholeness and midwifing healing, you can't help but develop a sense of awe and reverence for the inherent beauty and spirit of our fellow human beings. So at its best, in therapeutic touch we're dealing with something very spiritual.

To decide to become a practitioner of the technique is, in itself, to embark on a spiritual path. Healing, for instance, is the responsibility of the shaman in many cultures, which is the shaman's own personal spiritual path, and that's something we've almost lost in this culture. We've lost that sense of journeying along the spiritual path—at least our conventional healers have lost that sense and we don't think of going to medical school or nursing school as involving a spiritual path. But if we really want to facilitate genuine healing, that's exactly what we're doing.

That relationship of healing—any kind of healing—to a spiritual undertaking is a very interesting point.

It is. And it's important also for us to realize that we can learn to do therapeutic touch for each other. It's not something that's limited to doctors and nurses, since we all have the potential to heal in this way. That's the beautiful thing that Dr. Krieger did. She began to let people see that therapeutic touch is a natural human capability we possess for helping each other. Most of us have lost a sense of community when it comes to healing. We tend to think healing is something that takes place somewhere off in the hospital, separate from where we live. But of course it's not, and therapeutic touch is a way we can remind ourselves of that fact.

What is the primary goal of your research and work?

I really want to do something to empower people. I want people to realize that therapeutic touch is not just for special people to utilize. We all have to start recognizing our innate ability to help each other and we have to use it. That in itself would represent healing. For me to be able to help you, for instance—to interact with you in a healing way—is also healing to *me*. Now if each of us took that small step and began to see ourselves as healers, we'd also begin to see a healing of our community, our society, and our planet. And what could be more important than that?

14 | MANKIND: PROGRAMMED FOR RELIGION?

The late Dr. Helen Schucman is probably best remembered as the New York psychologist who spontaneously channeled *A Course in Miracles*. She underwent her first religious experience in a most unlikely place: She and her husband were riding a New York subway, having endured a fifteen-minute wait on a cold Manhattan platform. While being joggled by the train, she started noticing the shabby people riding the system. The scene was rather depressing, but then a blinding light consumed her and she lost contact with her environment. She saw herself within the light kneeling before somebody. The light grew more intense and she felt unconditional love emanating from it. Soon she found *herself* loving everybody including the grubby people on the train.

"I saw a great light and waves upon waves of love coming from it," she later explained, "and when I opened my eyes I loved everybody. Then everything disappeared... the feeling, everything."

Dr. Schucman immediately turned to her husband, a former library science student, and described her ecstatic experience. But he merely folded down the paper he was reading and said, "Don't worry about it. It's a common mystical experience. Don't give it another thought."

And with those pedestrian remarks, he went back to reading his paper.

The fact that Dr. Schucman had been plagued by both religious aspirations and conflicts throughout her life probably programmed her for this experience. (The fascinating story of her life and the reluctant creation of *A Course in Miracles* is told by Robert Skutch, who helped promote the scripts when they were written, in his short *191* book *Journey Without Distance.)* The fact remains, however, that many people experience brief ecstatic states in their daily lives. These types of occurrences have been called religious, cosmic, or mystical experiences. They represent the goal of some spiritual disciples, but everyday sorts of people commonly encounter them, too. There even seem to be two forms of the experience. In the first and predominantly pantheistic, the person loses self-identity and merges with nature or the entire universe. Becoming like a drop of water in the ocean is a common simile. The second type of cosmic experience is the impersonal mystical state, in which the person merges with other people. Both of these genres are typified by the sense of overwhelming love for God, nature, or each of its inhabitants.

Probably the first psychologist to focus scientific interest in these phenomena and catalogue such reports was, of course, William James (1842–1910). The philosopher/psychologist from Harvard based his famous Gifford Lectures to the University of Edinburgh on religious experiences. He had been previously drawn to the subject by the Stanford psychologist Dr. Edwin D. Starbuck, whose research focused on sudden religious conversion. The published version of these Gifford Lectures, *The Varieties of Religious Experience,* is chiefly concerned with conversion experiences and the subjective reports of great saints and mystics. The book is essential reading for everyone interested in spirituality or the psychology of religion.

THE NATURE OF MYSTICAL EXPERIENCES

The fact that such experiences could occur spontaneously and unrelated to religious conversion was documented in 1901 by the Canadian physician Richard Maurice Bucke (1837–1902) in his book *Cosmic Consciousness.* Bucke was drawn to the subject by his own mystical encounter, which he included in his book using the third person. The experience took place in England when the physician was thirty-six years old. He had spent the evening with friends reading poetry and was taking a cab back to his residence:

> They parted at midnight, and he had a long drive in a hansom. His mind deeply under the influence of the ideas, images and emotions called up by the reading and talk of the evening, was calm and peaceful. He was in

a state of quiet, almost passive enjoyment. All at once, without warning of any kind, he found himself wrapped around as it were by a flame colored cloud. For an instant he thought of fire, some sudden conflagration in the great city, the next he knew that the light was within himself. Directly afterwards came upon him a sense of exultation, of immense joyousness accompanied or immediately followed by an intellectual illumination quite impossible to describe. Into his brain streamed one momentary lightning-flash of the Brahmic Splendor which has ever since lightened his life; upon his heart fell one drop of Brahmic Bliss, leaving thenceforward for always an after taste of heaven. Among other things he did not come to believe, he saw and knew that the Cosmos is not dead matter but a living Presence, that the soul of man is immortal, that the universe is so built and ordered that without any peradventure all things work together for the good of each and all, that the foundation principle of the world is what we call love and that the happiness of every one is in the long run absolutely certain. He claims that he learned more within the few seconds during which the illumination lasted than in previous months, or even years of study, and that he learned much that no study could ever have taught.

While trying to describe the experience further, Bucke could say little more other than it was ineffable; for he could neither express his feelings in common language nor ever forget the episode. The experience prompted him to collect similar reports from the writings of famous religious readers, writers, and poets such as William Blake, Walt Whitman, and Edward Carpenter. The final section of his book recounts similar but "lesser" experiences from the lives of Spinoza, Pushkin, Thoreau and several people identified solely by their initials.

During the early years when Bucke, Starbuck, and James were conducting their research, it was not clear whether cosmic experiences were common or rare. The only thing clear was that the people reporting such encounters—separated both in time and place— seemed to be describing similar experiences. Their descriptions of the mystical state were so consistent that later philosophers had little problem typifying the "unitive" experience. Probably the best of these codifications was given in 1960 by the contemporary writer and philosopher W. T. Stace in his book *Mysticism and Philosophy,* where the cosmic experience is typified as follows:

1. The experience is characterized in terms of unitary conscious-

ness, in which the experiencer merges with God, nature, or *193*
  mankind.

2. The experience is nontemporal since the person's sense of time is overcome. Concern with the "real" world is lost simultaneously.
3. The recipient is left with no doubt concerning the realness or objectivity of the experience.
4. The person lucky enough to enjoy such an experience feels blessed by it, as if she or he were granted it.
5. The experiences seem to be intrinsically holy.
6. Since the mystical encounter cannot be explained psychologically, its core nature remains paradoxical.
7. The experience is ineffable since its essence cannot be captured in words.*

Even in the light of such analytical literature as Stace's commendable *Mysticism and Philosophy,* it is still nearly impossible to say whether such experiences are rare or common. This problem has been recently resolved, however, by research coming out of Great Britain.

Like most research into the metaphysical and the paranormal, the impetus for this work came from a single person. The late Sir Alister Hardy (1896–1985) was the chief zoologist on Great Britain's "discovery" expedition to the South Pole between 1925 and 1927. He later became Professor of Zoology and Oceanography at the University College of Hull, a post he held until 1942. During his tenure he was elected a fellow of the Royal Society. Professor Hardy took up similar responsibilities at Oxford University in 1946 and remained there until 1963, receiving his knighthood in 1957. It was in 1963 that he became Gifford Lecturer on Science and Religion at the University of Aberdeen. As the title of his post reveals, Professor Hardy was fascinated by religion, spirituality, and their interrelationship with science. So upon his retirement, he founded the Religious Experience Research Unit at Manchester College, where he set up offices in a private residence controlled by the institution. There he began collecting cases of spontaneous religious experiences reported from the general public.

---

* W. T. Stace's typography of the mystical experience is certainly not the last word on the subject, for other philosophers, including Bertrand Russell, have built similar characterizations.

194   Some of these early reports were included by Professor Hardy in his book *The Spiritual Nature of Man* published in 1979. In order to procure more representative examples of such phenomena, the Research Unit conducted a poll in 1975 on the religious experiences of the British public. The survey was orchestrated from Nottingham University by David Hay, who later reported the results in his own book *Exploring Inner Space,* which he provocatively subtitled *Is God Possible in the Twentieth Century?* (This volume was published in 1982.) It was pure good fortune that similar research was simultaneously being conducted in the United States by the National Opinion Research Center in Chicago. The findings of both polls were remarkably similar. When asked whether they had ever sensed some presence or power beyond themselves, thirty-five percent of the United States sample made the claim. The British public reported similar experiences thirty-one percent of the time. By using the proper statistical extrapolations, these numbers represent millions of people like you and me!

It is interesting to compare such figures with the results of a series of related Gallup polls. Surveys were conducted in the United States on the rate people report religious or conversion experiences in 1962, 1966, and 1967. The results of these studies suggest that between 20–41 percent of the American public have encountered such feelings!

It would not be prudent to spend further time on all these studies since a complete demographic analysis of these polls can be found in David Hay's book. Two findings from these surveys stand out, however, and deserve special comment. First is the fact that people from every possible religious persuasion — Jews, Catholics, Protestants and even self-proclaimed disbelievers — report such experiences. Also fascinating is that while churchgoers report them much more frequently, twenty-six percent of the British sample were not regular church people. It might also be mentioned that people predominantly experience religious episodes while by themselves, especially when suffering from emotional distress. Luckily, religious experiences seem to contain a healing essence and bring with them a sense of inner peace. Despite this characteristic, fifteen percent of the British respondents found such experiences frightening or troubling.

So what exactly is the mystical or religious experience? Do these occurrences represent genuine insights into the nature of the universe? Or are they simply hallucinations?

Several explanations for these ecstatic moments have been proposed over the years. Sigmund Freud was certainly interested in them, but considered "oceanic" feelings regressions (and therefore pathological episodes) in which the person—for psychological reasons—reexperiences the bliss of the prenatal womb. The fact that many people experience mystical rapture while suffering emotional distress supports such a theory, but what of the others? Mystical experiences tend to be triggered by external stimuli such as listening to music, contemplating nature, or engaging in passionate lovemaking. These are not usually considered frightening experiences! If we reject the facile psychological conceptualizations of the psychoanalysts, three explanations remain:

1. Religious and mystical experiences are genuine metaphysical moments by which we perceive reality's true nature.
2. Such encounters represent peculiar but probably nonpathological brain seizures, which result in intensely pleasurable and ecstatic experiences.
3. Such subjective phenomena possess no links to religion, but are completely neutral. We imbue them with religious connotations through our cultural and religious upbringings.

Good cases could be made for each of these conceptualizations, and I will leave it to the reader to choose whichever he or she prefers. But from my own reading of the literature, I would like to propose the following:

> *I feel that Mankind is programmed for religious belief and experience. There probably exists a center in the brain which is responsible for "coding" spirituality. This part of the brain is conceivably located in the older parts of the brain, from the standpoint of evolution, where it serves the purpose of regulating our perception of the universe's numinous nature.*

This suggestion may sound utterly fantastic, but I feel it can be supported by two lines of evidence. The first would be to show empirical evidence that such a neurological program exists for religious experience. I also believe that our religious beliefs possess a physi-

196 cal "energy" that can be gauged by standard scientific measurements.

According to the model I am proposing, cosmic and religious experiences represent this spiritual program functioning normally and efficiently within the brain. Now I could never prove such a concept and the skeptic could suggest that such experiences are merely seizures, perhaps linked to the brain's pleasure center. (Some epileptics, for example, report intense feelings of bliss before losing consciousness and/or entering seizure.) But my commitment to the "brain coding" model for spirituality is based on strong evidence that this center can function improperly—thereby inducing strange forms of spiritual and religious expression. So before proceeding further, I would like to take a protracted look at a peculiar phenomenon linked to epilepsy... the religious center within the brain "going haywire."

RELIGIOUS EXPERIENCE AND EPILEPSY

Religious beliefs seem to be intrinsic to mankind. Even prehistoric societies buried their dead, carefully preparing the bodies and even decorating them for their otherworldly journeys. In his pioneering book on primitive man, *The Golden Bough,* the great British anthropologist Sir James G. Frazer (1854–1941) suggested that religious belief resulted in part from dreams of the dead... thereby giving rise to the belief that the soul survives death. Other suggestions have been made during the century since the book was written.

Some early investigators posited that primitive man couldn't understand the natural world. Storms, whirlwinds, and other calamities were simply beyond his comprehension. So it was natural for our progenitors to create gods, demons, and finally religion to explain these wonders.

Working from the perspectives of folklore and early psychical research, the eminent British scholar Andrew Lang (1844–1921) postulated that ghosts really exist and that this phenomenon—coupled with the reality of the paranormal in general—gave rise to belief in immortality. This belief paved the way for the development of religion, a position he presented in his book *The Making of Religion* in 1898.

But probably the most current and controversial theory is that a propensity for religious belief is coded into the brain, as I suggested in the Introduction. Our nuministic sensibility and direct experience of the supernatural could be caused by unusual events taking place within its circuits. Religious beliefs would be a way some people try to *explain* these strange events.

Despite the sheer bizarreness of this notion, there is considerable evidence that the brain is a modulator for religious experiences. The phenomenon of sudden religious conversion, for example, is typical of such events within the brain and is a typical "symptom" of temporal lobe epilepsy. Small seizures in the temporal lobes can cause religiously toned hallucinations, which prompt the sufferers to believe they have a special mission in life mandated by God. These "revelations" sometimes bear little resemblance to the patient's prior religious beliefs or upbringing.

The fact that epilepsy is often complicated by "spiritual" insanity was well known to early experts on brain function. The phenomenon was often commented upon in books on the disorder written in the nineteenth century. The subject fell from grace for some reason until it reappeared by way of a comprehensive paper by Dr. Kenneth Dewhurst and Dr. A. W. Beard in 1970 in the *British Journal of Psychiatry.* Dr. Dewhurst was a research psychiatrist at the Littlemore Hospital in Oxford, while his colleague was an expert on psychological medicine at the Middlesex Hospital in London. The physicians reported on the most exaggerated form of temporal lobe epilepsy in their paper, in which remarkable religious visions and conversions were reported. Some of their cases read like testimonies from the Middle Ages, where self-perceived encounters with God, the Devil, and their minions seemed to be commonplace! The reports were collected predominately from Maudsley Hospital, where the patients had been examined and sometimes treated.

The first case presented in the paper concerned a 55-year-old male patient born in London in 1904. His religious background was typical for his Edwardian generation. He attended Sunday school for several years and considered himself a Christian, but religion was never really important in his life. The patient did, however, insist that his children go to similar classes. The gentleman's epilepsy first became obvious in 1941 when he suffered some noctural seizures while serving in the military. The seizures were presaged by a scream: his eyes would roll, his limbs would wave, and bladder control was lost. The seizures gradually became less frequent, but petit

198 mal episodes—brief moments of unconsciousness and lip-sucking—took their place. The religious aspects of his illness surfaced in 1955 during a severe depression when the patient was working as a bus conductor. One day he was overcome by feelings of extreme bliss and perceived himself to be in Heaven. He even reported his strange situation to his passengers. When he returned to normal, he tried unsuccessfully to explain his revelations to his wife, even though he couldn't recognize her. His mental state was so erratic that he was immediately hospitalized. During his stay, he claimed that he had literally seen God and could hear celestial voices and music. The patient was kept under observation for ten days, but even upon returning to normal, continued to believe in the reality of his experiences.

The patient remained stable for two years, but his seizures returned in 1958. These fits resulted in periods of elation in which he suddenly claimed that religion was false! Medical investigations conducted at Maudsley Hospital showed that the patient suffered from a lesion in his right temporal lobe. Some involvement from the left temporal lobe was also discovered and a left temporal lobectomy was performed in 1959 which cured the seizures. The gentleman remained religiously agnostic for the rest of his life.

A similar case originally reported from Maudsley Hospital concerned a thirty-five-year-old former Royal Air Force sergeant with a long history of epileptic seizures. These episodes commenced when he was a child, during which four grand mal seizures were recorded. It wasn't until he was twenty-four years old, however, that the condition returned. The patient reported that these seizures were sometimes presaged by the sensation that everything in his environment was unreal. He would then invariably stand up, bite his lips, clench his fists, and partially lose consciousness. Most of his seizures were minimal, with temporary loss of speech being their primary characteristic.

The patient's religious background was relatively unspectacular and typical for his times. While intensely religious in childhood, his spiritual preconceptions gradually ebbed and virtually disappeared by the time he reached twenty-one. But his involvement in religion returned when he was twenty-three years old and serving in the British military in Iraq. He suffered a minor seizure during this time, but didn't think much of it. A fortnight later, however, he strongly felt

God's presence and reality while strolling by his camp. This sense of deep spiritual reality reignited his religious commitments, but he soon lost his faith and backslid. The gentleman experienced a second religious conversion in 1954. The exact circumstances of the conversion are not spelled out by Drs. Dewhurst and Beard, but were sparked by two grand mal seizures which produced a florid religious psychosis in their wake. While at home recovering from the second seizure, the patient experienced a sense of unreality and saw a brilliant flash of light. The light represented God's presence (behind the sun) that was his simply for the asking. This sense of spiritual power soon gave rise to intense visionary experiences and schizophreniform delusions.

While being observed and treated at Maudsley Hospital, staff physicians determined that the patient's problems stemmed from discharges in the left anterior temporal lobe. A lobectomy was performed which cured the patient's epilepsy, but had little effect on his religious psychosis.

"Five months later," report Drs. Dewhurst and Beard, "the patient was still so involved in his psychotic experience that he had no interest in other topics. He completely believed in the validity of everything he had seen and heard during the acute phase, and specifically rejected the idea that the experience could have been the product of a disordered mind. He considered that he had received a message from God to mend his ways and help others, and the fact that he had been singled out in this way meant that he was God's chosen instrument.

"Twelve months after operation there were no new psychotic experiences to record, but his religious beliefs remained strong and he was attending church regularly. The patient had since remained fit-free."

Probably the most interesting case reported to the *British Journal of Psychiatry* concerned a Jewish patient born in 1920. This case is so fascinating because the subject never experienced grand mal seizures, remained sane, and constructively incorporated his conversion experience into his life.

The patient was described by his physicians as a shy, tidy, and meticulous homosexual. Born to an Orthodox Jewish family, he remained involved with his faith until he was seventeen years old. Even though he felt guilty over his religious lapses, the patient refrained from religious worship for several years before his dramatic

200 conversion. He suffered from petit mal seizures for most of his life, which manifested as brief losses of consciousness. His first conversion experience took place while he was being examined at St. Ebba's Hospital in England. Some tests of his brain function were being performed which employed photic stimulation. The stimulation resulted in a vision. The patient perceived himself flying a plane which brought him closer to God and he immediately became a Fundamentalist Christian. One night several months subsequent to the vision, he dreamt of the Crucifixion, which reinforced his religious beliefs. His third religious experience took place two months later while he was working. Heavenly hosts materialized before him which occluded his sight, even though he kept working at his job.

The patient had become fanatical by this time, but a friend moderated his religious beliefs and he became less dogmatic and entered the Methodist Church. Renewed medical investigations revealed that the patient suffered from a tumor in the right temporal lobe, but it was never removed. His seizures became less frequent over the years, but his religious commitments never changed.

"There was little diminution in his preoccupation with religion," report Drs. Dewhurst and Beard in their paper. "He soon brought any conversation round to a religious topic and frequently said that we must all believe in the Lord Jesus Christ. He had walked in the streets carrying a banner with the legend BE PREPARED TO MEET THY GOD, and he showed no ability to modify his conversation according to his company. He continued to believe that a religious meaning underlay ordinary events."

The British physicians report several other cases of sudden religious conversion linked to epilepsy in their pioneering paper, but space limitations preclude outlining them in depth. The following brief summaries cover the primary features of these cases:

- Their fourth case concerns a clerk who began suffering grand mal seizures in 1939. He discontinued taking medication to control them in 1954, which prompted his religious conversion—in which he perceived himself to be the Son of God gifted with both psychic and healing powers. A clinical electroencephalogram revealed an epileptic focus in the left temporal lobe.
- Drs. Dewhurst and Beard report on a female patient born in

1900 who suffered petit mal seizures every day. She began hearing the voice of God speaking to her when she was fifty-seven years old. A clinical electroencephalogram revealed idiopathic epilepsy (epilepsy of unknown cause) with a predominant focus in the right temporal lobe.

- The physicians' final case from Maudsley Hospital concerned a fifty-year-old Scot with little religious background. Upon recovering from a major seizure, the patient described himself as feeling "better than ever." He realized that he had a special mission from God to prove the Bible's truth. Medical tests revealed unusual electrical discharges from both the left and right temporal lobes. Further seizures later in life caused the patient to lose his religious commitment.

With such dramatic cases in the literature, it is a little puzzling that the phenomenon of sudden religious conversion is not more commonly discussed in books or surveys on epilepsy. Drs. Dewhurst and Beard failed to find the syndrome mentioned in some fifteen surveys of the literature published between 1954 and 1966. It is possible, of course, that these experts knew of such cases but failed to link these bizarre religious experiences with the epilepsy itself. Remember that even normal and healthy people experience sudden conversions and peak experiences, in which they become enveloped in unspeakable bliss!

Religiously toned visual experiences, delusions, and behavioral changes represent only a single component of the temporal lobe syndrome, however. The syndrome is really composed of three constituents, first outlined in the literature in the late 1970s by the late Dr. Norman Geschwind, then a psychiatrist with the Harvard Medical School in Cambridge, Massachusetts. His research into the temporal-lobe syndrome has been widely cited by other psychiatrists and neuropsychologists. In his book *The Social Brain: Discovering the Networks of the Mind,* for example, Dr. Michael S. Gazzaniga of Cornell University Medical Center offers the following description of the temporal lobe syndrome:

In reference to his esteemed colleague, Dr. Gazzaniga writes that "I would have been most skeptical of his account if I had not seen a case that exactly matched his description. This syndrome now has been reported several times. In its basic form, the brain injury causes

202 a deepening of religious conviction, a desire to write extensively *(hypergraphia)*, and the performance of bizarre sexual activity. There is no a priori reason I know of why affecting one of these behaviors ought to affect the other two!

"The reality of the syndrome is not amusing. Of interest here is the religious behavior aspect of the syndrome. Not only is conviction deepened, but the form it takes becomes erratic and the person switches from one belief to another rapidly and without apparent cause."

A similar description is given by Dr. Robert G. Feldman of the Boston Veterans Administration Medical Center in his textbook *Neurology: The Physician's Guide:*

> Based on a century of clinical observation, there evolved a literature describing a series of personality characteristics that were seen in the *interictal state* of patients with TLE [temporal lobe epilepsy]. These characteristics are of three categories. First, there are manifestations of an overconcern with details, a tendency to give equal weight to all experiences. In the retelling of experiences there is overinclusiveness, endless iterations of small details and circumstantiality. There is a tendency to write down events, keep diaries and journals or scrapbooks of important experiences. Second, there are manifestations of emotional intensity. Life events are seen in a cast of unusual moral or cosmic importance. The patients often become very religious or adopt deep philosophic frames. They are often intensely moral, although perhaps on a personal idiosyncratic framework. They may have a tendency to develop deep and lasting emotional states (anger, elation, and depression). Third, they are usually hyposexual.

Note that there is some disagreement over the sexual expression of the temporal lobe syndrome. Some experts comment on the lack of sexual urges in these people—perhaps linked to a deficiency in blood-borne precursor hormones that stimulate the production of sex hormones. (Such a finding has been made by physicians researching temporal lobe epilepsy.) But other researchers point to hypersexuality as a component of the disorder. Some psychiatrists, on the other hand, report bizarre sexual expression exhibited by temporal lobe epileptics—such as cross-dressing and fetishism.

Probably the most unusual aspect of the syndrome is the temporal

lobe epileptic's propensity for compulsive writing, or hypergraphia. *203*
The content of the scripting is usually meaningless, pedestrian, or
painfully redundant.

Dr. Stephen Waxman, of Boston City Hospital, and Dr. Norman
Geschwind published a classic paper on this phenomenon in the July
1974 issue of *Neurology,* in which they describe seven typical cases.
One of them concerned a thirty-four-year-old patient who suddenly
complained of headaches and gastrointestinal problems. Brain
abscesses were discovered and surgically repaired by his physicians,
but the patient later developed symptoms of left temporal lobe problems. The epilepsy was treated with standard drugs. But even though
the drugs kept the seizures under control, bizarre changes in the gentleman's behavior soon manifested. He developed an intense fascination with religion and began suffering grand mal seizures. He completely lost interest in sex and began offering his services to religious
organizations. The patient spent considerable time writing extraordinary sermons, trying to find "hidden meaning" in life's pedestrian
events. Some words of the sermons were written completely in capital
letters, while the writings themselves included frequent digressions.

A second case reported by Drs. Waxman and Geschwind concerned a temporal lobe epileptic who suffered from a compulsion to
produce metaphysically oriented poetry.

Despite the obviousness of such symptomology, the existence of a
clearly defined "temporal lobe syndrome" has not gone unchal-
lenged within psychiatry. Some experts in the field point out that the
temporal lobe syndrome isn't commonly seen in a random cross section of temporal lobe patients, while similar symptoms crop up in
other forms of psychopathology. In other words, since the temporal
lobe syndrome isn't specific to epilepsy, there is little evidence that
these behaviors—hyperreligiosity, hypergraphia, and unusual sexuality—specifically link to brain misfiring. Other psychiatrists and
neurologists point out that since standard medication fails to change
these symptoms, they are probably behavioral and not neural in
nature.

The fact that there do exist specific behavioral concomitants to
temporal lobe epilepsy was, however, formally documented in 1977
despite this formidable debate. This research emerged from the
National Institutes of Neurological and Communicative Disorders and

204 Stroke in Bethesda, Maryland. It was published in the *Archives of Neurology* in 1977.

As part of this project, Dr. David M. Bear and Dr. Paul Fedio evaluated the personality characteristics of forty-eight temporal lobe epileptics by subjecting them to intense psychological probes. Some of these patients suffered from problems in the right temporal lobe, while the others suffered from left temporal disorders. Their scores and ratings on the personality inventories were then compared to a control group, carefully matched to the epileptics by chronological age, education, and other demographic features. What the researchers found were specific differences not only between the epileptics and the controls, but even between right and left temporal lobe epileptics. Some of these differences were reminiscent of the religious predispositions outlined in earlier psychiatric literature. Right temporal lobe epileptics, for instance, reported more periods of elation and a sense of "destiny" in their lives. Such personality characteristics could be precursors to the religious conversions reported by Dr. Kenneth Dewhurst and Dr. A. W. Beard in 1970.

The left temporal lobe subjects shared some of these same characteristics. "Left temporal patients were identified with a sense of personal destiny and a concern for meaning and significance behind events," report the researchers. "Related items emphasized powerful forces working with one's life... and the need for sober intellectual and normal self-scrutiny..." Both groups reported a consistent interest in religious and philosophical issues more extreme than seen in the control group.

While perhaps a far cry from the specific temporal lobe syndrome described earlier by Dr. Gazzaniga and Dr. Geschwind, it certainly seems clear that religious belief is partially exaggerated in some epileptics... and that these propensities somehow link up with events occurring within the brain's convoluted circuitry.

So what do these findings mean? Do they imply that religious revelations, peak and cosmic experiences, and even spiritual beliefs are delusions? Perhaps faulty beliefs produced by the brain for some unknown reason? Or is there a deeper meaning to the epileptic's fascination with the spiritual world?

Several experts on epilepsy and neuropsychology have taken up the challenge of these issues.

Probably the most cynical interpretation of the temporal lobe syn-

drome is offered by Dr. Michael Gazzaniga in his book *The Social* 205
Brain. His belief is that the epileptic focus somehow interferes with
the patient's critical sensibilities, so that (s)he begins to uncritically
incorporate strange beliefs—such as religious doctrines—into his or
her everyday life. Critical thinking becomes difficult and the patients
eventually immerse themselves into magical ways of perceiving the
world. Dr. Gazzaniga expands this line of speculation by suggesting
that brain malfunction virtually explains the rise of religion throughout mankind's history.

Skepticism of religion plays a related role in the viewpoints promoted by Dr. Kenneth Dewhurst and Dr. A. W. Beard. They point out
in their *British Journal of Psychiatry* report that several celebrated
religious figures of the past were probably epileptic—including
everyone from St. Paul to St. Teresa of Avila. St. Paul's conversion on
the road to Damascus is especially suspect, they point out, since he
saw a bright light and fell when the conversion took place. The
British investigators suggest that religious conversion is a purely neu-
rocognitive phenomenon. Discharges within the brain inhibit the critical capacities of the epileptic's higher brain functions, which serve
as the seat of mankind's critical thinking. The conversion is not the
direct result of the discharge, though. Changes of consciousness
result from these neural firings, which excite more primitive and
emotional levels of the brain. In order to find "meaning" in these
sudden changes in consciousness and perception, the epileptic draws
upon his early religious background. In other words, the epileptic
erroneously interprets his strange experiences as the result of some
external force—such as God or Jesus—and not as events produced
within his or her own body.

Drs. Dewhurst and Beard trace this conceptual model back to the
speculations of the great British brain expert Sir Hughling Jackson
(1835–1911), who first proposed them in 1876. They report that some
evidence supporting Jackson's theories can be found in their own
data. Most of the conversions they studied were experienced by people with some prior religious exposure. Their religious preoccupa-
tions were probably revitalized by their epilepsy, not created by the
seizures.

Probably the most moderate explanation for the temporal lobe syndrome was proposed by Dr. Norman Geschwind, who first isolated
and described the purported temporal lobe syndrome in the 1970s.

206 The late Dr. Geschwind rejected the criticism that the syndrome's characteristics—hyperreligiosity and so forth—were psychological in nature. Stress certainly doesn't cause the epileptic to become religious, the psychiatrist points out, since similar stress is typical of several diseases in which hyperreligiosity plays little role. On the other hand, the psychiatrist didn't believe that the syndrome was solely produced by the epilepsy itself. Since temporal lobe behaviors increase when the epilepsy is medicated, the source of these behaviors is probably psychologically intrinsic to the patient. Dr. Geschwind suggested that some sort of disinhibition in the limbic system could be the source of the behavior. (The limbic system is a collection of organs within the brain that regulate our emotional responses—from bliss to rage. These organs lie deep within the brain.)

"We seem to be faced with a paradox, but I believe that it can be resolved simply," explained the psychiatrist in a paper on temporal lobe epilepsy he published in 1983 in the journal *Epilepsia:*

> My speculation is that this syndrome is the result of the presence of an intermittent spike focus [unusual electrical discharges] in the temporal lobe. The presence of the focus leads to an alteration in the responsiveness of the limbic system, so that the patient's emotional responses are altered in characteristic fashion, i.e., there is heightened emotional response to many stimuli, and diminished sexual responsiveness. The spike focus can, of course, also behave in such a fashion as to produce epilepsy. Either or both of these can occur independently.

One result would be extreme emotional responsiveness to ordinary events taking place in the world. Believing himself chosen by God for some mission could be the way the epileptic makes sense of this exaggerated responsiveness. The religious visions of the temporal lobe epileptic probably result from electrical stimulation of its temporal cortex and these hallucinations, too, become incorporated into this search for meaning.

While each of these explanations for the temporal lobe syndrome *could* be partially correct, I would like to repropose the model I briefly suggested in this chapter. This theory departs radically from the reductionistic viewpoints typical of contemporary psychiatry and neuropsychology. As I said earlier, *perhaps the brain is specifically coded for religious experience, so that mankind possesses a natural method for directly perceiving the spiritual world.* Such a focus would be similar to those complexes within the brain which regulate vision and speech. What is seen in temporal lobe epilepsy is some sort of *malfunction* in this brain center or complex. In people with a preexisting brain problem such as temporal lobe epilepsy, stimulation of this center causes spiritual or "religious" insanity. But in normal people, *perhaps this center regulates a deep connection between the brain and its capacity to establish contact with the spiritual world.*

This theory might sound fanciful, but recent evidence has emerged from the field of genetics suggesting that the brain is specifically wired for religious belief. This new evidence indicates that there exist deep connections mediating between the brain, genetics, and mankind's religious nature.

This research has been conducted in Great Britain by the iconoclastic psychologist Dr. Hans Eysenck and in this country by investigators with the University of Minnesota. Both projects looked at the religious views, sentiments, and behaviors of identical twins reared separately from birth or early childhood. Both research teams found that such people often "develop" surprisingly similar religious sympathies and even behaviors—i.e., a propensity toward observing the Sabbath or taking the Bible literally. Now these findings lead us to ask the following question: For what purpose is mankind neurologically and genetically *programmed* for religious belief? My private suspicion is that, through the process of evolution, mankind has developed the capacity to directly perceive the spiritual world. We wouldn't have this power unless the brain were sensitized to its existence. But like so many organs of the body, this part of the brain could have fallen into dormancy through lack of use. It may come into play today only when people experience "mystical states" ... or when it goes berserk due to epilepsy or a related dysfunction.

THE POWER OF PRAYER

Now I said earlier that our religious beliefs possess an "energy" that can be measured by science. I was referring to the power of prayer. Does prayer really work? There is considerable experimental evidence that it can, and it is to this subject I would like to turn.

208   Perhaps I should begin this section with some words of wisdom from the great scientist who said, "The great thing is to pray, even if it be in a vague and inarticulate fashion."

These words weren't delivered from a pulpit or by a television evangelist, but by John William Strutt (1842–1919), the third Lord Rayleigh, the recipient of the Nobel Prize in physics in 1904. While granting that the Victorian era was less secular than our own materialistic times, it is still interesting that intellects such as Lord Rayleigh publicly promoted the benefits of prayer.

No less celebrated a Victorian scientist was Sir Francis Galton (1822–1911), whose pioneering research led to the emergence of both eugenics and criminology as scientific disciplines. Back in 1883 he pondered the issue of prayer in his *Inquiries into Human Faculty and its Development.* The great scientist was especially fascinated by the subject of petitionary prayer—i.e., those prayers we sometimes offer to help other people cope with their personal problems. Since he was primarily an experimentalist, Galton made the following remarks in his book.

"It is asserted by some men," he wrote, "that men possess the faculty of obtaining results over which they have little or no direct control, by means of devout and earnest prayer, while others doubt the truth of this assertion. The question regards a matter of fact, that has to be determined by observations and not by authority."

It is clear from this remarkable passage that Galton considered the "power of prayer" to be a testable hypothesis. When the sick are prayed for, he wondered, do they really tend to recover more readily in response? .

The problem Galton confronted was not in properly framing his question, but in determining a method by which to test it. He finally decided to make a survey on the possible physical benefits of petitionary prayer. He figured that people who are commonly prayed for, such as sovereigns, should have longer life spans than lay people. So he collected mortality figures for selected monarchs in Europe and compared them to a random sample of Great Britain's public. There was little difference in the statistics, and in fact, the monarchs tended to die younger than the commoners! Sir Francis wasn't daunted by these results, and proceeded to collect life span figures for British clergymen—people for whom prayer played a frequent role in their daily lives—and compared them to figures collected for people such as lawyers and physicians. Since, again, there was no evidence that *209* the clergy outlived the secularists, Galton became disillusioned with studying prayer.

The experimental scientists of today would probably not be impressed by Galton's research, especially since the eminent researcher never bothered to directly experiment with the possible power of prayer. But the public statements and research of such great scientists as John Strutt and Sir Francis Galton prove an important point: The power of prayer need not rest simply on faith, since it may be a scientifically testable possibility.

Research into any scientific issue can be approached in two ways: either by collecting case histories which support the issue, or by directly testing your theory. So to begin this inquiry into the power of prayer, let us start by looking at some cases bearing on the subject. Does petitionary prayer work?

An excellent case that points to this possibility was reported by John Fagan, a middle-aged Glasgow dockworker, who first became ill in April 1967. On the morning of April twenty-sixth he awoke feeling ill and began vomiting blood. He was immediately taken to Glasgow Royal Infirmary, where he underwent two days of medical tests. The results were hardly encouraging, and on May fourteenth his physician performed stomach surgery—carefully concealing from his patient that his problem was stomach cancer. The surgical examination revealed just what the physician most feared: The cancer had spread from the stomach into the colon and couldn't be completely removed. So when the surgery was over, the doctors could only tell Mrs. Fagan that her husband couldn't survive much longer. They suggested that she help to get her husband's personal affairs in order, and told her that John would die within six months.

John Fagan's condition progressively worsened over the next six months, and by the end of summer, he could hardly eat. The poor man was deteriorating so badly that his wife took him back to the hospital just before Christmas. During this stay, his physicians found that secondary malignant tumors were spreading throughout the patient's body. Since there was simply nothing further they could do for the dying man, they merely sent him back home to die.

Because he was completely bedridden, Mr. Fagan received precious few visitors during these crucial months. His only spiritual comfort came from Father John Fitzgibbon, the associate pastor of the

210 Church of Blessed John Ogilvie in Glasgow. The priest realized that his parishioner was dying and even administered the last rites when Fagan took a turn for the worse in January. But two months later, five friends of the dockworker's decided that prayer might work where medicine had failed. So on the evening of March 5, 1968, these friends formed a prayer group by his bedside and petitioned for John's full recovery. Since they were Roman Catholics, they naturally proceeded to pray in that tradition. Catholic belief teaches that prayers can be answered by holy people from the past, people still interested in our physical and religious well-being. So the prayer group directed their prayers to the Blessed John Ogilvie, a seventeenth century Scottish martyr.

It should be mentioned that at this time, prayer was probably the *only* thing that could have helped the patient. When the Fagans' doctor visited the sick man the next day, he was shocked by John's condition. He briefly examined the patient and then left, somberly telling Mrs. Fagan that he would return in a few days to sign his death certificate.

The "miraculous" cure of John Fagan became evident the next day, merely two days after the prayer group's bedside ministrations. After falling into an unusual and deep sleep, he woke that morning feeling much better and even asked for food! Even though he had taken practically no nourishment in weeks, now he was hungry. Fagan further told his wife that his pain was gone and he didn't display his daily habit of regurgitating. Within a matter of weeks, in fact, John Fagan made a complete recovery from his spreading and obviously terminal cancer.

The case seemed too good to be true, so in October 1967, Roman Catholic authorities in Glasgow began looking into the incident. Father Thomas Reilly of the Church of Blessed John Ogilvie organized the investigation by collecting all of Fagan's medical records. These records and reports were subsequently turned over to a panel of prominent physicians, who deliberated for two years before concluding that the cure was medically inexplicable. Only a medical expert from Glasgow University harbored any doubts about the cure, and his objections were countered by the other panel members.

By this time the miraculous cure of John Fagan had become a cause célèbre in Scotland, so in 1971 Catholic officials in Rome sent their own medical experts to examine the case. Professor Livio

Capacacci was a specialist in gastroenterology with the University of *211* Rome, where he served as a medical advisor to the Vatican. He gathered together a second panel and cooperated with Father Reilly in reevaluating the case... from start to finish. Dr. Capacacci was specifically concerned with the possibility that Fagan's recovery was caused by spontaneous remission, the cure of a secondary disease unrelated to the original cancer, or some other "natural" explanation. When these possibilities were finally rejected by the panel, John Fagan's cure was proclaimed miraculous by the Vatican on February 12, 1976.

But what caused the cure? Was it produced by the supernatural intercession of the deceased John Ogilvie, which was the common belief of the Glasgow prayer group? Or did their *intention* to heal their friend through prayer *directly* cure him? In other words, did some sort of mysterious power generated by the prayer interact with the dying man's body, gradually making it whole?

This second possibility seems more scientifically feasible, since similar remarkable cures have been reported from other than Catholic traditions. Such cases are related so commonly that in 1983 a British physician published a special study of them. The *British Medical Journal* isn't exactly the place you'd expect to find a paper on the power of prayer, but the December issue (a Christmas special), included a fascinating article on the subject contributed by Dr. Rex Gardner. Dr. Gardner is currently a consultant obstetrician and gynecologist at Sunderland District Hospital. Before taking up that position, he worked as a missionary physician.

The incident that first sparked Dr. Gardner's interest in the benefits of prayer took place in 1970, when he treated the captain of the Girls' Brigade at Enon Baptist Church in England. The poor girl suffered from a large varicose vein which obstinately refused to heal. It had become so ulcerated that, every morning, she had to redress the puss-soaked bandages binding the lesion. Since the prescribed medical treatments weren't helping, Dr. Gardner didn't know what else to tell his patient, who soon took the situation into her own hands. She decided to have a prayer service said for her when the church scheduled its next prayer meeting. Dr. Gardner didn't object to the plan, but he warned the patient that he was pessimistic about whether prayer would help her. He even accompanied her to the meeting, but told her that the lesion would require skin grafting even if the ulcer

212 *were* healed. With these frightening words still resonating in her ears, the prayers were offered for her recovery by the parishioners of the church.

The prayer service heralded the gradual cure of the captain's ulcerated leg. When she woke the following morning, the lesion was dry and healthy skin had inexplicably started to cover it. Only a single small spot in the ulcer continued to secrete a discharge. This recalcitrant spot bothered the captain throughout the following week until a brigade lieutenant scheduled a meeting with the church's pastor. She explained that she should have participated in the prayer meeting, but hadn't, and she desperately wanted to help the other girl. The pastor and the young lady immediately visited the patient, where they performed the laying on of hands. The little ulcerated spot spontaneously healed during the session, and no skin grafts were necessary.

Dr. Gardner seemed almost reluctant to report the case in his *British Medical Journal* paper since it was so bizarre, but he explained that the case rested on his personal documentation.

Because of this personal experience, Dr. Gardner decided to find other cases of miraculous cures resulting from prayer and witnessed by physicians such as himself. Some of these healings represented instances of distant healing, which he found especially provocative.

One of these fascinating cures was reported to the British physician in January 1975 from Wales. The exact location and the name of the patient were withheld by Dr. Gardner, who personally contacted the physicians who treated the case. The patient was a physician-in-training who contracted meningococcal septicemia with meningitis, a serious infection of the membranes covering the brain and spinal cord. The patient's condition worsened by the time she was diagnosed the next day as having a malignant form of epidemic cerebrospinal meningitis. This syndrome is usually fatal and the hospital treating her had never seen a remission or cure. News of the patient's condition soon spread, however, and religious groups held meetings in four Welsh cities that evening to pray for her. The petitioners asked not only that she recover, but that the cure would be complete and perfect.

These prayers were said at roughly 8:30 in the evening, and the doctors noted that the patient began to improve at the same time.

An eyewitness to the cure later explained to Dr. Gardner that, beginning that evening, "there was a sudden improvement in her con- *213* dition, though it was four days before she regained consciousness. [The] physicians were unable to explain how her chest x-ray film, which had shown extensive left-side pneumonia with collapse of the middle-lobe, could, forty-eight hours later, show a normal clear chest."

This statement perhaps suggests that, somehow, the prayers speeded up the body's normal healing process. But there was a side effect to the healing which made it even more spectacular. One serious result of the infection was the formation of a blind spot in the patient's left eye, caused probably by a hemorrhage. The blind spot was extremely conspicuous, and it was the opinion of the hospital opthamologist that it would cause permanent eye damage. But whatever "power" healed the patient knew its business, for the eye healed completely... to the surprise of the specialist, who knew of no similar reported case.

A second case study pointing to the regenerative power of prayer was reported to Dr. Gardner by some Lutheran nuns in Damstadt, Germany. This "miracle" occurred when the Evangelical Sisters of Mary were building a chapel in 1951. One of the order fell onto a freshly cemented floor, broke through it, and landed on a wooden beam. The result of the mishap was a compound pelvic fracture. The nun was rushed to the local hospital, where the physician told the nuns that their Sister would require traction for several weeks. The doctor was therefore dismayed when the Sisters took the injured woman back to their residence, where they prayed for her and offered the laying on of hands. Despite the warnings of the doctor, the Sister was healed in two weeks without any medical treatment, whereupon she revisited the hospital so that the physician could document the cure. Dr. Gardner personally contacted the witnesses and learned that, when the healing was completed, the fortunate Sister was able to walk without any trace of a limp.

The three cases summarized in this report represent a brief sample of Dr. Gardner's accounts. The original paper he offered in the *British Medical Journal* included seven case studies. It is the physician's opinion that while the existence of the miraculous can never be proved, these cases represented true medical mysteries. "The adjective 'miraculous' is, however, permissible," he concludes in his paper, "as a convenient shorthand for an otherwise almost inexplicable healing which occurs after prayer to God."

214   Similar case studies could be summarized from a large body of literature—both religious and medical. But summarizing these cases wouldn't serve any real purpose. The existence of merely a single miraculous cure through prayer should be enough to make the student of religion take the practice seriously. The skeptic, however, will probably never be convinced by such accounts, even if the evidence were to become ironclad. I learned this lesson myself through personal experience in 1984, when I sent a copy of Dr. Gardner's paper to a well-known skeptic with a Ph.D. in physiology. I was curious to hear his response to the report, since he was a complete skeptic of the paranormal. After he read the report, he told me that the British physician's cases could be explained by spontaneous remission. When I then asked him how such remissions could heal broken bones or cure incurable conditions, he simply refused to reply. He countered by saying that the only proof of the miraculous would come when God helped somebody to regrow an amputated leg! When I suggested that perhaps healing through prayer might have certain limitations, he merely scoffed.

It is for this reason that the power of prayer can best be proved not by collecting field reports, but by conducting rigorous experimental research. Few people know that several experiments into the healing power of petitionary prayer have been designed and implemented, often with surprising results. Some of the first work was reported in the early 1950s by Rev. Franklin Loehr. Rev. Loehr was originally a chemical engineer but turned to religion and founded the Religious Research Foundation in Los Angeles. Later he became familiar with Dr. J. B. Rhine's research into extrasensory perception and psychokinesis (mind over matter) at Duke University, which he felt might explain the sometimes remarkable effects of prayer. Since he remained a scientist by training, Rev. Loehr decided to see whether prayer would help plants to grow, and soon conducted several experiments to prove his case. His basic design entailed asking his subjects to pray over seeds and seedlings, while using identical plots for his controls. The results of these studies demonstrated that the prayed-for plants usually grew better, so in 1959 he published his famous little book *The Power of Prayer on Plants*. This slim volume included the results of nine hundred trials, eight thousand measurements, and the efforts of one hundred and fifty subjects.

The 1950s also hosted the experimental work of Dr. William R. *215* Parker of Redlands, California. Dr. Parker was interested in whether personal prayer could be used for self-healing, so he organized prayer groups in the area. By personally working with these groups, the professor taught his subjects *how* to pray and met together with them to discuss the results. Dr. Parker documented some impressive cures of such conditions as stuttering and migraine, but it is hard to determine what exactly produced the changes. These disorders tend to be caused or exacerbated by psychological factors so his study showed only that prayer is a powerful psychological tool for healing. But he failed to show that the results were the outcome of a special or unique power of prayer.

Despite the shortcomings of the Redlands project, Dr. Parker's *Prayer Can Change Your Life* became a classic in the 1950s and still remains a thoughtful study on the personal benefits of prayer. More rigorous research into the power of prayer had to wait until the 1960s, when the first double-blind experiment was executed.

It has never come clear what factors originally led Dr. C. R. B. Joyce (a psychopharmacologist) and Dr. R. M. C. Welldon to carry out their unusual work. It seems likely that their interest in spiritual healing was sparked by the Church of England, which began studying the powers of religious healing in the 1950s. (Their favorable report was issued in 1956 and suggested that physicians and clergymen should work together to heal the sick.)

Whatever the case may be, the two researchers soon began their work at London Hospital Medical College, where they focused on several patients suffering from either rheumatoid arthritis or emotional problems. The subjects were matched in pairs by such factors as chronological age and clinical diagnosis, and the names of only one member from each group were sent to prayer groups in several British cities. The other members of the matched pairs served as the controls for the study. The prayer groups were instructed to pray by contemplating a passage from the Bible while mentally focusing on the patients. For some inexplicable reason, however, the groups were not told to pray specifically *for* the patients. This peculiarity may explain why the results of the project were mixed, for the two researchers failed to find that the prayed-for patients fared any better than the controls.

216   The most important upshot of the study, however, was that it encouraged a pediatrician in the United States to replicate the experiment, and his results were considerably more impressive.

Dr. Platon J. Collipp was chairman of the pediatric department of Meadowbrook Hospital in New York when he decided to design and implement research into prayer. The original impetus for his research came after he read a report by Drs. Joyce and Welldon in a 1965 issue of the *Journal of Chronic Disease.* Since Dr. Collipp *was* a specialist in pediatrics, he focused his own experiment on childhood leukemia, a terribly serious and usually fatal disease.

Dr. Collipp initiated his research project by requesting several colleagues to supply him with personal information on their young leukemia patients. The result was that he was able to employ eighteen patients receiving similar forms of chemotherapy for his study. Needless to say, the children never knew that the study was in progress nor their role in it. Dr. Collipp then recruited ten families living in Washington state, who were instructed to pray for ten randomly selected children. These families were not instructed in any particular form of prayer, and the study lasted for fifteen months. What the New York physician hoped to find was that the prayers either helped the children overcome the disease or extended their lives.

The results confirmed Dr. Collipp's hopes and served as a lesson for the medical establishment. By the end of the project, only two of the eight control children had survived the leukemia. The medical histories for the prayed-for children stood in striking contrast, with eight of them still surviving. Even though the subject population was small, the difference in survival rates reached statistical significance. The results prompted Dr. Collipp to write in his report for the *Medical Times* that "among the plethora of modern drugs, and the increasing ingenuity of our surgeons, it seems inappropriate that our medical literature contains so few studies on our oldest, and who knows, most successful form of therapy." He concluded by saying that "every physician has prescribed this remedy and every physican has seen it succeed."

The problem with this research into the power of prayer should be clear to the reader, however. The studies designed in England and the United States relied on small sample sizes, and Dr. Collipp was forced to admit in his report that his subject population was so small that it nearly prevented him from employing the proper statistical *217* measurements on his data. Perhaps it was for this reason that his research was greeted by no fanfares from medical circles or by the press. But these experiments remain, even today, a most interesting and curious footnote in medical research's history.

That situation may have also resulted from the social climate in the 1960s, when conventional (allopathic) medicine was king and the general public its obedient serf. With the rise of holistic medicine in the 1970s, however, even many conventional physicians began looking toward such procedures as biofeedback and related mind/body tools with some interest. Books such as Dr. Kenneth Pelletier's *Mind as Healer Mind as Slayer* summarized the purely scientific/psychological theoretical basis for holistic medicine, while otherwise conventional people began looking to Eastern religions to reinvigorate their spiritual lives. With such a revolutionary milieu evolving within popular culture, research into the power of prayer was bound to make a comeback. The breakthrough finally came when the usually staid *Medical Tribune* published the following story by Maury Beecher headlined in its January 8, 1986 issue:

3 CARDIOLOGISTS REPORT PRAYERS FOR THEIR PATIENTS ARE 'ANSWERED'

The article began by saying, "Should cardiologists pray for their patients? Three leading cardiologists do—and they recommend the practice to their colleagues."

The basis for the story stemmed from a paper delivered shortly before to the American Heart Association by Dr. Randolph Byrd, a cardiologist (then) with San Francisco General Hospital, during their convention in Florida. Dr. Byrd had long been a devout Christian and decided to experiment with the power of prayer. What resulted was the most elaborate and significant study ever conducted on the subject.

Dr. Byrd began his experiment by programming a computer to match a group of cardiac patients, for whom prayers would be said, to a similar group of control subjects—i.e., other heart patients whose problems would receive medical treatment but no spiritual healing. The computer program eventually selected 192 experimental patients and 201 controls, whose medical progress Dr. Byrd studied for sever-

218 al months. So that the experiment would be properly controlled, Dr. Byrd did not personally pray for the patients, but recruited religious practitioners throughout the country to help him. These people came from Protestant and Catholic backgrounds, and were simply given the names of the people they were to help. Dr. Byrd asked the participants to offer their prayers every day. While many of the volunteers prayed privately, some of the others formed small prayer groups. The experiment lasted close to a year, and the final results looked rather clear-cut. Dr. Byrd reported three major effects resulting from the study to the convention:

- While sixteen of the control patients needed to take antibiotics to treat illness-related infections, only three of the experimental subjects needed them during the course of the experiment.
- Even though eighteen of the controls suffered from pulmonary edema (water in the folds of the lungs), the complication was reported for only six of the prayed-for patients.
- While twelve of the control subjects required intubation due to their cardiac problems, not a single patient in the experimental group needed help in breathing.

Each of these findings reached statistical significance, the measure scientists use to determine if an experimental finding is due to chance or not. Dr. Byrd's first two findings would only result from chance *once* every one hundred times the experiment was run. His third effect would be expected to result from chance with odds of twenty to one.

Even more surprising than these results were the reactions to the study published by the *Medical Tribune* in the same issue. While the publication didn't formally poll its readership, the editors collected several statements from other physicians in support of the Byrd study. The well-known physician and writer Dr. William Nolen, a strong critic of religious healing, told reporters from the *Chicago Sun-Times* (who reported the *Medical Tribune's* story) that "it sounds like this study will stand up to scrutiny." This statement stood in stark contrast to the opinions he expressed in his scathing book *Healing: A Doctor in Search of a Miracle,* in which he labeled spiritual healing worthless.

There has, in fact, been rather little public criticism of Dr. Byrd's *219* study from within the medical community. (Some spokesmen from organized religion have responded to it, fearful that people will misinterpret the study and renounce religion if their prayers remain unanswered.)

Despite his careful methodology, Dr. Byrd later encountered serious problems publishing his study in a mainline medical journal. It finally appeared in print in 1988 in the *Southern Medical Journal.*

Scientific experiments and field investigations into the mystery of prayer seem impressive, but more research is obviously called for— using more subjects, more physicians, and looking into more and more biological disorders and sicknesses. The religious skeptic will, however, probably never be satisfied with the evidence, but in time, this extreme position will fade like a Cheshire cat's smile. It will evaporate when more people start employing prayer to heal themselves and those they love. When people start personally experimenting with prayer and objectively seeing its effects, the purely scientific debate over the power of prayer and religious belief will become less and less important. What will remain a mystery is the *extent* to which prayer and faith can cure, and whether certain forms of prayer work better than others.

That day may be coming soon.

It is certainly possible that the power of prayer has little to do with religion. Perhaps it is merely a potential each of us possesses similar to psychokinesis, the mind-over-matter power studied by parapsychologists.

I personally tend to disagree with this claim. I have spent years working in the field of parapsychology. During that time I have observed and conducted several psychokinesis experiments. The typical laboratory subject possesses this power in a rudimentary form, so weak that it takes complicated equipment—such as rapid oscillators—to detect it. This force strikes me as a different type of power than that unleashed through prayer. But even if the power of prayer does not prove that mankind is by nature religious, it shows—if nothing else—that we can connect to other people in ways science cannot explain. This finding leaves open the possibility that life on this plan-

220 et is interconnected and directly wired to the fabric of reality. Isn't this one of the primary messages of religion in general?

So as I have said repeatedly in this chapter, mankind seems programmed for spirituality. Simply stated, if there were no truth in religion, there would be no reason for the brain to be coded for it. So let us learn to use the power of faith... both by healing our inner wounds and by praying for those we love. Each of us has this responsibility to make the world a better place.

The following bibliography includes books on inner healing and self-development reflecting the subjects covered in this book. I have not tried to compile a comprehensive guide, since the collected literature on these topics is enormous. I have instead selected a sampling of books under eight subheadings. The criteria for inclusion consisted of three factors: (1) the book had to be in print or available at public libraries, (2) consist in part of instructions for self-help, and (3) be written by an expert in his or her field. A few exceptions were made to these principles and have been noted in the descriptions.

I. STRESS MANAGEMENT

McCullough, Christopher J. and Robert Woods Mann. *Managing Your Anxiety: Regaining Control When You Feel Stressed, Helpless and Alone.* Los Angeles: Jeremy P. Tarcher, 1985.

Written in part by a professional psychotherapist, this book focuses on the nature of situational and state anxiety. The entire second part of the book outlines, in considerable detail, a self-care program including relaxation exercises, methods for dealing with emotional distress, overcoming inappropriate learned responses, relaxation, assertiveness training, and so forth. It also includes an excellent suggested reading list.

Pelletier, Kenneth R. *Mind As Healer Mind As Slayer.* New York: Dell, 1977.

Anyone interested in psychoneuroimmunology—how the mind influences the immune system—should begin with this classic, which includes detailed information on stress and the body. The first three parts of the book contain a sophisticated overview on the psychology and psychodynamics of stress and its relation to disease. The fourth part consists of three chapters which discuss specific stress reduction strategies: meditation, visualization, biofeedback, and autogenic training. While not specifically written as a self-help guide, the reader will find many suggestions for stress reduction in the discussions.

Pelletier, Kenneth R. *Healthy People in Unhealthy Places—Stress and Fitness at Work.* New York: Dell, 1985.

Since most people find that their work is a primary stressor, it isn't surprising that Dr. Pelletier would write a book on. the subject! This volume served as the focus for the interview with the psychologist printed earlier in this book. Not only does Healthy People in Unhealthy Places outline stress problems and toxic hazards in the workplace, it is especially strong in directing the reader to health promotion programs (Chapter 4) and resources (Appendices A and B).

Rathus, Spencer A. and Jeffrey S. Nevid. *BT—Behavior Therapy.* Garden City, New York: Doubleday, 1977.

An excellent introduction to one of psychology's strongest tools. Behavior modification might give rise to visions of brainwashing, mind control, and laboratory rats. In reality, most stress reduction strategies are based on simple behavioral therapy. This book has been written for the general public by two psychologists who explain BT techniques and offer suggestions for their use in everyday life. Included are procedures for relaxation, body work, self-reward, overcoming phobias, better sleep habits, assertiveness training, better sex, weight reduction, overcoming smoking, and other specific issues.

Sheehan, David V. *The Anxiety Disease.* New York: Bantam, 1986.

This short paperback is described by its publisher as "new hope for the millions who suffer from anxiety." There isn't much new in the book, but it is a handy guide on the subject that will provide the reader with some important insights into the problem. The second part of the book is specifically devoted to treatment, but is not as systematic as the McCullough and Mann book.

II. PERSONAL GROWTH

(The literature on humanistic psychology, personal growth, and spiritual development is so vast that no short bibliography could ever do it justice. I have therefore suggested in this section a handful of books reflecting different approaches to these subjects.)

Fields, Rick., et. al. *Chop Wood, Carry Water: A Guide to Finding Spiritual Fulfillment in Everyday Life.* Los Angeles: Jeremy P. Tarcher, 1984.

While lacking the depth of many books on spirituality, this lovely and engagingly produced book compiled by the editors of the *New Age Journal* explains how to find spiritual fulfillment in everyday life. For those readers nostalgic for the 1960s this volume is virtually a *Whole Earth Catalogue* on inner growth. It covers virtually every aspect and approach to spiritual growth: from interpersonal relationships to sex, spirituality in the workplace to detachment from material goals, and from earth consciousness to strategies for inner peace. Every section has suggested reading lists, resources, lists of pertinent organizations, and photographs.

Ferrucci, Piero. *What We May Be: Techniques for Psychological and Spiritual Growth.* Los Angeles: Jeremy P. Tarcher, 1982.

Dr. Ferrucci is a follower of Dr. Roberto Assogioli, who developed psychosynthesis as the practical side of transpersonal psychology. This book outlines Assogioli's system. Each section focuses on direct applications for the reader. These include both body and mind exercises for several life problems: inner focusing, body awareness, drawing exercises for self-understanding, contacting inner selves, visualization, dealing with aggression, self-examination, and other topics. While sometimes a bit esoteric, the book contains a plethora of information on self-discovery.

Gendlin, Eugene I. *Focusing.* New York: Bantam, 1981.

One of the truly unique books on inner development. Dr. Gendlin is a Chicago psychologist who has developed a fascinating technique for identifying life-problems and their possible solutions. The key is on how the body responds (by subtle changes) when a problem is correctly spotted and the right solution mentally proposed. Dr. Gendlin's system is not as well-known as it should be and represents a concise and practical program for self-help.

Goldberg, Philip. *The Intuitive Edge: Understanding Intuition and Applying It in Everyday Life.* Los Angeles: Jeremy P. Tarcher, 1983.

What is intuition? Nobody really knows, but it is a potential each of us possesses and should be able to employ in daily life. This readable book discusses research on intuition from Jungian psychology to experimental work. Chapters 8 and 9 outline a program for developing intuition and learning to rely on it. These suggestions are highly concrete and Mr. Goldberg—a writer with a degree in industrial psychology—explains the ways they can be used in daily problem solving.

Hay, Louise L. *You Can Heal Your Life.* Santa Monica, California: Hay House, 1984.

Since Dr. Hay was interviewed in this book, it certainly seems appropriate to include her best-known book, which showed up on *The New York Times* best-seller list when it was originally published. The book outlines New Thought/self-help philosophy in extremely simple terms. While written from a specific spiritual tradition, the volume could serve as a good starting point for readers just beginning to delve into the metaphysical literature on personal growth. The chapters focus on Dr. Hay's personal philosophy and how it applies to daily living. The book is especially good in showing readers how to identify life-problems and the resistance we have to change.

Harman, Willis and Howard Rheingold. *Higher Creativity.* Los Angeles, California: Jeremy P. Tarcher, 1984.

Partly written by an acknowledged leader in the human potentials movement, this is the best book I'm familiar with on the psychodynamics of creativity. Exploring everything from intuition to dream work, suggestions for using creativity in everyday life are incorporated into the chapters. An excellent guide to a complicated yet provocative subject which doesn't oversimplify it.

Houston, Jean. *The Possible Human: A Course in Extending Your Physical, Mental, and Creative Abilities.* Los Angeles, California: Jeremy P. Tarcher, 1982.

Dr. Jean Houston, too, is certainly one of this country's pioneers in the study of self-transformation, inner development, and the psychology of consciousness. Explicitly written in the form of a self-help manual, this detailed book describes techniques for better body connection, sensory enhancement, brain power, memory usage, and creativity. The book's drawback (not lost on several of the reviewers who criticized it upon publication) is that some of the exercises are *too* detailed. Following them requires frequent referral to the book, thereby compromising the reader's concentration.

Tart, Charles T. *Waking Up: Overcoming the Obstacles to Human Potential.* Boston: Shambhala, 1987.

One of my personal favorites, Dr. Tart's book is filled with uncommon wisdom on the human condition, but still manages to convey these insights in a chatty, informal manner. The book is nearly seductive, in the positive sense of the word. It begins by outlining the psychology of personal growth, explores the nature of reality, and then proceeds to offer the reader a program for functioning more effectively by virtue of these insights. The second part of the book is primarily based on the psychological/spiritual system for personal growth created by the eccentric spiritual teacher G. I. Gurdjieff, which Dr. Tart has simplified from its nearly incomprehensibly esoteric form.

III. STRATEGIES FOR OVERCOMING DISEASE

Benjamin, Harold H. with Richard Trubo. *From Victim to Victor: The Wellness Community Guide to Fighting for Recovery for Cancer Patients.* Los Angeles, California: Jeremy P. Tarcher, 1987.

Santa Monica, California, has long been the home for the Wellness Community, founded by Dr. Benjamin for the holistic treatment of cancer. While never suggesting that proper medical treatment should be ignored, Dr. Benjamin is a follower of the theory that emotional factors complicate the disease. This book outlines a self-care program for cancer patients and their families: psychologically dealing with the disease, strategies for fighting for recovery, coping with friends and family, and visualization exercises for overcoming sickness. Also included is a complete description of the Wellness Community itself.

Chopra, Deepak. *Creating-Health: Beyond Prevention, Toward Perfection.* Boston: Houghton Mifflin Co., 1987.

Written in a popular first-person style, this volume offers a nice introduction to the principles of holistic health. Dr. Chopra discusses the various conditions and diseases caused by stress and related emotional factors, such as hypertension, heart disease, cancer, drug dependency, gastrointestinal problems, sleep and sexual disorders, and on and on. Next he outlines a curriculum for total health based on standard holistic principles: self-consciousness, egogratification, the power of the mind, diet, and so forth. The last part of the book covers the use of meditation for better health, especially TM[tm]. Not as sophisticated as his *Quantum Healing* (reviewed below), it is still enjoyable in its own right.

Chopra, Deepak. *Quantum Healing: Exploring the Frontiers of Mind-Body Medicine.* New York: Bantam, 1989.

Reading this book encouraged me to meet and interview Dr. Chopra. In a sense it takes over from where Dr. Chopra's autobiography, *The Return of the Rishi: A Doctor's Search for the Ultimate Healer* (Boston: Houghton Mifflin Co., 1988), finished, but familiarity with that book is not necessary. This sophisticated book outlines the new frontiers of psychoneuroimmunology. It is filled with the writer's own case studies of patients who recovered from serious illness through better thinking, coping strategies, and holistic stylings. The book imparts a great deal of medical and research information at the same time, which will appeal to the scientifically oriented reader.

Jaffe, Dennis T. *Healing from Within: Psychological Techniques to Help the Mind Heal the Body*. New York: Simon and Schuster, 1986.

Books on the role of psychological factors in health seem to be proliferating. It's a popular topic these days, but this six-year-old book remains one of the best. Dr. Jaffe is a psychologist and *Healing from Within* was a *Medical Self-Care* magazine book award winner. It is written (predictably) from a more psychological than medical perspective, and is more self-care oriented than Dr. Justice's book on the same subject (see below). The entire third section of the book is concerned with coping and recovering strategies in the face of sickness: relaxation exercises, information on biofeedback, learning to control self-defeating behavior, establishing contact with our inner healer, etc.

Justice, Blair. *Who Gets Sick: How Beliefs, Moods, and Thoughts Affect Your Health*. Los Angeles, California: Jeremy P. Tarcher, 1988.

Written by a psychologist at the University of Texas Health Service Center, *Who Gets Sick* is an excellent guide to the literature on psychoneuroimmunity. Dr. Justice has extracted hundreds of experiments from the psychological and medical literature on the subject, which he presents in a concise and well-organized manner. His comprehensive reference lists are worth the price of the book. While not written expressly as a self-help manual, the four sections comprising Part 5 fulfill this function with guidelines on the power of faith, love, and self-action in the face of disease.

Roud, Paul C. *Making Miracles: An Exploration into the Dynamics of Self-Healing*. New York: Warner Books, 1989.

The term "exceptional patient" refers to those people who beat the odds either by recovering from life-threatening diseases or outliving their physicians' predictions. Dr. Roud, a psychologist in Massachusetts, offers his readers profiles of eleven such people who overcame—psychologically, medically, or both—conditions ranging from cancer, to spinal disease, to schizophrenia. Each study is followed by Dr. Roud's own insightful observations on the psychodynamics behind the recoveries and scientific research pertinent to them. While not a self-help guide, the book should bolster the morale of the reader facing serious illness.

Simonton, O. Carl, Stephanie Matthews-Simonton and James Creighton. *Getting Well Again: A Step-by-Step Self-Help Guide to Overcoming Cancer for Patients and Their Families.* Los Angeles, California: Jeremy P. Tarcher, 1978.

What needs to be said about this book, probably the most famous volume on self-healing ever written? Dr. Simonton is an oncologist who first brought organized medicine's attention to the role visualization can play in fighting cancer. The book followed the publicity and controversy sparked by his claim. Especially notable is a discussion on correct and *incorrect* visualization strategies. Such related issues as coping with residual fear, building family support systems, and overcoming resentment when illness strikes are not sidestepped either. Still a classic and probably always will be.

ALSO RECOMMENDED:

The books of Norman Cousins and Dr. Bernie Siegel are so well-known that they need no protracted comment. Mr. Cousins tells the story of using humor and psychology to overcome ankylosing spondylitis (a serious spinal condition) in his *Anatomy of an Illness As Perceived by the Patient: Reflections on Healing and Regeneration* (New York: W. W. Norton, 1979). The similar story of his recovery from a coronary is offered in his *The Healing Heart: Antidotes to Panic and Helplessness* (New York: W. W. Norton, 1983). His most recent book concerns his work at U.C.L.A. putting his insights to work. *Head First, The Biology of Hope* (New York: Dutton, 1989) is an enjoyable autobiography, which includes a great deal of information regarding U.C.L.A. research on psychological factors in medicine.

Dr. Bernie Siegel's first book on the exceptional cancer patient was *Love, Medicine and Miracles* (New York, Harper and Row, 1986). I personally prefer his sequel *Peace, Love and Healing: Bodymind Communication and the Path to Self-Healing: An Exploration* (New York: Harper and Row, 1990) which is a more personable look at exceptional patients and the lessons Dr. Siegel has learned from them.

IV. DEALING WITH DEATH AND GRIEF: DYING

Buckman, Robert. *I Don't Know What to Say... How to Help and Support Someone Who Is Dying.* Boston: Little, Brown, 1989.

This excellent book is designed as a guidebook for readers serving as support persons for friends and relatives facing death. Included is detailed information on talking with the dying, the psychology of death, and for saying good-bye. While not himself drawn to religion, a chapter is included on the spiritual dimensions of death and dying, offered by a clergyman and colleague of the writer's.

Carroll, David. *Living with Dying.* New York: Paragon House, 1991.

Even though this book is not written by a professional clinician, it can be recommended without hesitation. It is a virtual encyclopedia of death-related information. The focus is on helping the reader face death constructively, with sections included on: talking about death, the stages of death, caring for the terminally ill, patient rights, children and death, care of the dying child, home health care for the seriously ill, hospice care, and preparing for life's end. A worthwhile endeavor that should enjoy a wide readership.

Richards, Larry and Paul Johnson. *Death and the Caring Community.* Portland, Oregon: Multnomah Press, 1980.

Unlike the other books summarized in this section, *Death and the Caring Community* approaches the subject from a strictly religious framework. It basically argues that Christians have a responsibility to minister to the dying and that such work leads to spiritual growth. Liberally highlighted with citations from the Bible, the book recounts the true-life stories of people who grew psychologically by helping the dying and includes a thirty-four-page section on "Training for Caring." It also includes a first-rate bibliography of books, films, and video-tapes on death. While the book's strongly sectarian approach will not be for everyone, it nonetheless contains some excellent information.

Roth, Deborah and Emily Le Vier (editors). *Being Human in the Face of Death.* Santa Monica, California: IBS Press, 1990.

Edited by two professional social workers, this short book has been issued by a small California publisher currently issuing a series of books on spirituality, death, and bereavement. Each of the book's first eight chapters concerns a different psychological response to death. The second part is devoted to the care giver's own needs and mental health resources. Metaphysics and death is the third topic covered, and the book concludes with a workbook for the care giver. This section offers writing and other exercises by which readers can connect with their own reactions to life's end.

White, John. *A Practical Guide to Death and Dying: Conquering Fear and Anxiety Through a Program of Personal Action.* Wheaton, Illinois: Theos, 1988.

Written before books on death and bereavement became so popular, John White's book draws upon his long association with the human potentials movement Mr. White offers exercises and insights on facing our fears of death, learning meditation to deal with them, growing old, and planning for death intelligently. While some of the material reads like padding, other sections offer the evidence for life after death... one of the few books on the subject to tackle this issue. Mr. White correctly realizes that familiarity with this large body of evidence, in itself, can help people overcome their fears.

ALSO RECOMMENDED:

The books of Dr. Elizabeth Kübler-Ross have been bypassed since they are so famous. Nor are they particularly meant for self-improvement or spiritual growth. Her five major volume's include her best-selling *On Death and Dying* (1969), which outlines the five "stages" of life's final transition—even though independent research has failed to confirm such a progression. This book was followed in 1974 with *Questions and Answers on Death and Dying*. *Living with Death and Dying* (1981) concerns care for the dying, with special emphasis on using drawings to help people confront and interpret their emotions, a procedure Dr. Bernie Siegel was later to use with his patients. *Working it Through* was published in 1982 and concerns working with the terminally ill in small groups. Dr. Kübler-Ross later turned to the special problems of children facing death and her work with them is chronicled in *On Children and Death*, published in 1983. All of these titles were issued in hardback by Macmillan and Co. and in paperback by Collier Books.

I noted earlier that IBS Press in Santa Monica is publishing a series on death, dying, and grief recovery. Included in this series are *Gifts for the Living: Conversations with Care Givers on Death and Dying*, edited by BettyClare Moffatt, and *The New Age Handbook on Death and Dying* by Rev. Carol W. Parrish-Harris. IBS Press can be contacted by writing to: 744 Pier Avenue, Santa Monica, California, 90405.

V. DEALING WITH DEATH AND GRIEF: AFTERWARD

Kutscher, Austin H., et. al. (editors). *For the Bereaved: The Road to Recovery*. Philadelphia, Pennsylvania: The Charles Press, 1989.

Dr. Kutscher (himself a two-time widower) and his associates have been busy with their New York-based Foundation of Thanatology editing textbooks on the subject. This anthology is their first attempt to share the fruits of their wisdom with the general public. The volume helps the reader understand grief from the standpoint of religion, psychiatry, and social work. Short sections cover special problems encountered in specific types of grief: over the deaths of children, suicides, spouses, and so on. Excellent chapters are included on the psychological benefits of funerals, mourning rituals, grief and health maintenance, conflicts over remarriage, and financial management. While the chapters are not of equal quality, the book might be a good starting point for the bereaved reader.

Lukas, Christopher and Henry M. Seiden. *Silent Grief: Living in the Wake of Suicide.* New York: Bantam, 1990.

Suicide is one of the leading causes of teenage death in the United States, and a common cause of mortality in adults. The effects of suicide on surviving family members can be devastating. Such families can be consumed by guilt and unable to find support from their embarrassed friends. This book has been written by one such survivor in collaboration with a professional clinician. The first part recounts Mr. Lukas's own problems dealing with his mother's suicide. Part Two describes the psychology of suicide and the type of reactions seen in the surviving families. More self-help in orientation is Part Three on "Giving Help and Getting Help," which concerns strategies for families facing suicide and offering support to others. The book ends with a complete list of suicide support groups in the United States and a short bibliography.

O'Connor, Nancy. *Letting Go with Love: Grieving Professional.* New York: Bantam, 1989.

For the reader who wants a once-over-lightly book on grief, this slim volume by a professional psychologist should fit the bill. For such a relatively short book (168 pages of primary text), Dr. O'Connor packs a great deal of information into her chapters. She outlines grief styles, the stages of grief, and then like most books on the subject, focuses on special grief problems: reacting to the death of spouses, parents, children, infants, friends, and suicides. Listings for grief-related service organization and similar resources are included.

Rando, Therese A. *Grieving: How to Go on Living When Someone You Love Dies.* Lexington, Massachusetts: Lexington Books, 1988.

This volume by one of this country's leading experts on bereavement could be called "everything you ever wanted to know about grief." It is extremely comprehensive, combining information of psychological studies of bereavement with concrete suggestions for self-recovery. As with the Lukas and Seiden and O'Connor books listed in this section, Dr. Rando organizes her volume around specific types of grief problems. The most reader-oriented part of the book is Part IV on "Resolving Your Grief," which outlines a practical grief recovery program for the bereaved person. One chapter (15) gives extremely specific recommendations for grief recovery, while the following chapter discusses the promises and *limitations* of bereavement processing. The book is long and sometimes bogs down, but it represents a solid resource guide on the subject.

Staudacher, Carol. *Beyond Grief: A Guide for Recovering from the Death of a Loved One.* Oakland, California: New Harbinger Publications, 1987.

Most books on grief read somewhat the same, but Carol Staudacher's book is different, for it offers sophisticated insights into the psychodynamics behind the grief process. The reader comes to really understand why we grieve and the specific causes of our sometimes irrational behavior in the face of death. The first fifty pages of the book on the grief experience itself is the best explanation of bereavement I have ever read. From these promising beginnings, Ms. Staudacher discusses the loss of spouses, parents, children, and the special problems posed by sudden death. The last large section of this book contains information on procuring help and starting a support group. Supporting bereaved friends is discussed toward the book's close. *Beyond Grief* is a perfect blend of objective information and self-help instruction.

Tatelbaum, Judy. *The Courage to Grieve: Creative Living, Recovery, and Growth Through Grief.* New York: Harper and Row, 1984.

Had I not liked this relatively compact book so much, I wouldn't have pushed to interview Ms. Tatelbaum for *Science of Mind* magazine. The book's focus is on the stages of grief and the ways we work through bereavement. While discussing grief processing, Ms. Tatlebaum draws on her gestalt psychology background to show that specific exercises exist for grief recovery. Some of these are offered in her chapter "Helping Ourselves with Grief: Creative Survival." Most books on grief seem content with helping readers resume their previous level of functioning, but this one goes further... by showing how bereavement can be used for personal and spiritual growth.

VI. SPIRITUAL PARENTING

Armstrong, Thomas. *The Radiant Child.* Wheaton, Illinois: Theos, 1985.

A somewhat uneven book, the writer—who holds a doctorate from the California Institute of Integral Studies in California—explains the transpersonal inner world of children. He surveys the child's world within the context of (heavily Jungian) psychology, metaphysics, and mythology. Next he explores the world of children's subjective experience, including the psychic and mystical encounters they so often report. More reader-oriented is Chapter 9, "Helping Children on Non-Ordinary Levels," which echoes some of what Dr. Keith Harary said in his interview. Probably the most useful sections of the book, however, are its three appendices. The first is an annotated bibliography of transpersonal children's literature. The second is a general reading list of books on children and their higher nature, while the last concerns resources for transpersonal children's studies. These excellent guides make up for the text's deficiencies.

Carroll, David L. *Spiritual Parenting.* New York: Paragon, 1990.

Written by the same journalist whose *Living with Dying* was highly recommended in Section IV, this volume is for people with strong spiritual beliefs who want to impart them to their children. It is written from a strictly nonsectarian standpoint and draws upon recommendations from several religious traditions. The first three parts of the book summarize some basic child-rearing strategies. The fourth, fifth, and sixth sections concern creating a spiritual environment in the home, teaching children moral values, and the use of prayer and meditation in child-rearing. The book also includes detailed recommendations for children's literature that imparts moral or spiritual messages. A very good introduction to a very difficult subject, capably written and presented.

Skutch, Judy and Tamara Cohen. *Double Vision.* Berkeley, California: Celestial Arts, 1986.

This book is not exactly on spiritual parenting as such. It is a double autobiography, first by Judy Skutch (who was instrumental in publicizing and promoting *A Course in Miracles*), whose daughter Tamara was highly psychic in childhood. It is placed in this section because Tamara looks back on her childhood in her contribution and explains everything her mother did wrong in dealing with her—not to mention the parapsychologists who were called in to investigate the case. An honestly written book, it will serve as an object lesson for parents facing psychically gifted children.

Tanous, Alex and Katherine F. Donnelly. *Is Your Child Psychic?* New York: Macmillan, 1979.

While not a particularly good book (and in places downright bad), this volume will hopefully educate parents on children and their sixth sense. Part IV is devoted to information on testing children for psychic powers, but whether the results or failures of such ESP games could emotionally harm children is not considered. Read this book for the information it contains, not for the writers' opinions.

Young, Samuel H. *Psychic Children.* Garden City, New York: Doubleday, 1977.

This volume is everything the Tanous and Donnelly book should have been but wasn't. Specific topics on childhood psychism—ESP, psychokinesis, premonitions, past-life recall, and sensitivity to other worlds—receive chapters side-by-side with four elongated case studies. The real crux of the book is Chapter 9, "Growing Up Psychic."

Mr. Young takes the middle path on the subject: We should neither glorify nor invalidate children when they claim psychic experiences. He also shows how parents can explore their children's experiences in a calm, objective but nonthreatening gamelike atmosphere. Some of the best writings to be found on this provocative subject.

VII. THE POWER OF TOUCH

Cohen, Sherry Sued. *The Magic of Touch.* New York: Harper and Row, 1987.

Written by a professional journalist, Ms. Cohen's book might be a good starting place to study touch and its multifaceted dimensions. The book was published as part of Harper and Row's *New Ways to Health* series. While not a terribly sophisticated book, it takes brief looks at the following: loving touch, therapeutic touch, acupressure, massage, reiki, rolfing, chiropractics, the Feldenkrais method, reflexology, and so forth. Strategies for using touch in everyday life are given in Chapter 7, but Ms. Cohen should have resisted the temptation to call her final chapter "Finishing Touches." Too cute for words, but it leads to a fine guide to where touch and massage can be learned.

Older, Jules. *Touching Is Healing: A Revolutionary Breakthrough in Medicine.* Chelsea, Michigan: Scarborough House, 1982.

Much more sophisticated than the Cohen book reviewed previously, psychologist Jules Older canvasses scientific and psychological research on touch, while recounting the story of his own experiences using touch for psychological healing. Surveyed is the vast literature on touch and birthing, massage, holistic health, medicine, and other topics. The book's only problem is Dr. Older's dislike for the paranormal and the suggestion that touch contains a bioenergetic component. A large section of Chapter 9 ridicules valid scientific research on the paranormal effects of touch on plant growth, blood chemistry, and other phenomena. Dr. Older doesn't even offer a satisfactory reason for rejecting these findings, saying merely that "I reject the evidence because I do not believe it." This is supposed to be science? So skip this nonsense and enjoy the other chapters and the book's fine detailed bibliography.

Krieger, Dolores. *Living the Therapeutic Touch.* New York: Dodd, Mead and Co., 1987.

A sequel to her previous *Therapeutic Touch* (Englewood Cliffs, New Jersey: Prentice-Hall, 1979), Dr. Krieger spends the first 125 pages of this book discussing touch within the context of yoga, creativity, parapsychology, and evolution. Her message is that since everyone has the power to heal through touch, contemporary society should nurture this power. For some strange reason, the rest of the book consists of nineteen appendices on using therapeutic touch in childbirth. Why this information wasn't structured into a readable chapter is beyond me.

Macrae, Janet. *Therapeutic Touch: A Practical Guide.* New York: Alfred A. Knopf, 1988.

For readers specifically interested in techniques for therapeutic touch, this short ninety-one-page monograph should suffice. Dr. Macrae is both a nurse and a therapeutic touch practitioner and explains the techniques in easy to follow detail. The book is richly illustrated, so it is difficult not to understand the procedures. The last chapter discusses the self-transforming effects of practicing therapeutic touch. Highly recommended as a study guide on the subject.

VIII. MUSIC, HEALTH, AND GROWTH

Green, Barry and W. Timothy Gallwey. *The Inner Game of Music.* Garden City, New York: Doubleday, 1986.

Mr. Green has been the principal bass player with the Cincinnati Symphony for many years while W. Timothy Gallwey has written several previous books on the "zen" or inner games of golf and tennis. Together they show how musicians can improve their performance skills through psychological exercises. This book is not really for the everyday person, but can be profitably used by musicians both amateur and professional.

Halpern, Steven with Louis Savary. *Sound Health: Music and Sounds That Make Us Whole.* New York, Harper and Row, 1985.

The interview with Mr. Halpern included in Part I of the present book will give the reader a good idea of his book's scope. It is probably the best introduction on physical and mental health benefits/issues linked to music outside of the professional literature on neurophysiology and music therapy. The book is divided into four parts; the first three are devoted to the effects of music on the body, mind, and spirit. The fourth part lists resource guides for the reader who wants to put this material into action. Mr. Halpern and his coauthor distill a great deal of technical information in this book, and their efforts certainly pay off. Both readable and sophisticated, with just the right blend of science, speculation, and a hint of metaphysics.

Lingerman, Hal A. *The Healing Energies of Music.* Wheaton, Illinois: Theos, 1983.

While awfully metaphysical in places (in the *worst* sense of the word), this book was written as a guidebook for using music constructively in everyday life. Chapters are included on finding the best music for yourself, using music for everyday chores, selecting music for the home, and other subjects. His guide to the music of the great masters is sometimes simplistic and highly subjective, but never misleading. All in all, this is a fun book to read, especially for beginning music lovers who want a basic introduction to the classics and the practical use to which it can be applied.

Scarantino, Barbara Anne. *Music Power.* New York: Dodd, Mead and Co., 1987.

Written by a professional music therapist, this book explains the fundamentals of understanding and appreciating music. Chapter 3 turns to the physiological and biological effects of music on human cells, plant growth, muscle strength, brain waves, and other physiological variables. Not sidestepped is the way some music, especially when played too loud, can hurt instead of heal us. Addiction to rock music is discussed in this section. The book is especially strong on how to use music in everyday life: for relieving hostile emotions, in conjunction with stress-management programs and other pertinent situations. Over forty pages list suggested music, both popular and classic, to play for exercise and other purposes: from studying and learning to better sex.

I. HUMANISTIC AND TRANSPERSONAL PSYCHOLOGY

Applebaum, Steven A. *Out in Inner Space*. Garden City, New York: Anchor/Doubleday, 1979. A wonderfully appealing firsthand exploration of the "growth" therapies by a psychoanalyst.

Grof, Christina and Stanislav. *The Stormy Search for the Self: Understanding and Coping with Spiritual Emergency*. Los Angeles, California: Jeremy P. Tarcher, 1990.
A quirky book on personal growth through "transformational crisis," In other words: What to do if you go bonkers while looking for God and self.

Grof, Christina and Stanislav (editors), *Spiritual Emergency*. Los Angeles, California: Jeremy P. Tarcher, 1989.
Writings on the psychological and spiritual problems that can crop up while traveling the cosmic path.

Hardy, Jean. *A Psychology with a Soul: Psychosynthesis in Evolutionary Context*. New York: Penguin, 1990.
An introduction to the transpersonal psychology of Roberto Assogioli.

Hoffman, Edward. *The Right to Be Human: A Biography of Abraham Maslow*. Los Angeles, California: Jeremy P. Tarcher, 1988.
A comprehensive biography of Abraham Maslow, the founder of humanistic psychology.

Ornstein, Robert E. *The Psychology of Consciousness*. New York: Penguin, 1986.
The book that first popularized—and simplified—the concept of left/right brain hemisphere function and how to make use of this lateralization.

Tart, Charles T. (editor). *Transpersonal Psychologies*. Novato. California: Psych Processes, 1983.
The classic book on the psychological systems imbedded in the world's great spiritual traditions.

Wilson, Colin. *New Pathways in Psychology*. New York: Taplinger,

1972.

A history of humanistic psychology and the post-Freudian revolution.

II. HEALING AND SELF-DEVELOPMENT

Achterberg, Jeanne. *Imagery in Healing Shamanism and Modern Medicine.* Boston: Shambhala, 1985.
An intelligent and sophisticated discussion of the role imagery plays in healing, from shamanism to contemporary cancer and immunological research.

Carlson, Richard and Benjamin Shield (editors). *Healers on Healing.* Los Angeles, California: Jeremy P. Tarcher, 1989.
Over thirty healers—metaphysical, medical, religious, psychological, and so on—discuss their art.

Hunt, Morton. *The Compassionate Beast.* New York: Morrow, 1990.
What psychology is discovering about compassion, our inner drive toward goodness.

Mitchell, Janet Lee. *Conscious Evolution.* New York: Ballantine Books, 1989.
The relationship of ESP to the evolution of human consciousness.

Storr, Anthony. *Solitude: A Return to the Self.* New York: Ballantine Books, 1989.
The constructive use solitude can play in our lives, written by a Jungian therapist.

Tatelbaum, Judy. *You Don't Have to Suffer: A Handbook for Moving Beyond Life's Crises.* New York: Harper and Row, 1989.
A handbook for learning techniques and strategies for confronting life's inevitable crises.

Weill, Andrew. *Health and Healing.* Boston: Houghton and Mifflin, 1983.
A reevaluation of holistic practices from homeopathy to psychic healing by one of pop culture's leading iconoclasts.

III. EVERYDAY MYSTICISM

Cohen, J. M. and J. F. Phipps. *The Common Experience.* Los Angeles, California: Jeremy P. Tarcher, 1979.

A good introduction to the study of religious experience.

Greeley, Andrew M. *Ecstasy: A Way of Knowing.* Englewood Cliffs, New Jersey: Prentice-Hall, 1974.

A fine study on the practical side of the mystical sense, written before the author became so famous!

Johnson, Raynor. *Watcher on the Hills.* London: Hodder and Stoughton, 1959.

One of the classics on mystical experiences reported by the general public.

Laski, Marghanita. *Everyday Ecstacy.* London: Thames and Hudson, 1980.

Described (correctly) by the publisher as "some observations on the possible social effects of major and minor ecstatic experiences in our daily lives."

Sinetar, Marsha. *Ordinary People As Monks and Mystics.* New York: Paulist Press, 1986.

Looks at people who have found spiritual satisfaction in their ordinary lives.

IV. DREAMWORK

Gackenbach, Jayne and Jane Bosveld. *Control Your Dreams.* New York: Harper and Row, 1989.

Learning to create lucid dreams for fun, personal transformation, and physical health.

Garfield, Patricia. *Creative Dreaming.* New York: Ballantine Books, 1985.

Controlling your dream life and the lessons we learn from it.

Kelsey, Morton. *Dreams: The Dark Speech of the Spirit.* Garden City, New York: Doubleday, 1968.

The role dreaming has played in Christian thought, history, and belief.

La Berge, Stephen. *Lucid Dreaming.* Los Angeles, California : Jeremy P. Tarcher, 1985.

The story of the writer's research on lucid dreaming.

Sanford, John A. *Dreams: God's Forgotten Language.* New York: Harper and Row, 1989.

The psychological and spiritual messages encoded into our night-time reveries.

Signell, Karen A. *Wisdom of the Heart.* New York: Bantam, 1990.

Dreamwork for women from a Jungian perspective.

Ullman, Montague and Nan Zimmerman. *Working with Dreams: Self-Understanding, Problem-Solving, and Enriched Creativity Through Dream Appreciation.* Los Angeles, California: Jeremy P. Tarcher, 1985.

Forming and working with small dream groups.

V. MEDITATION AND VISUALIZATION

Carrington, Patricia. *Freedom in Meditation.* Garden City, New York: Anchor/Doubleday, 1978.

What research is telling us about meditation, and how it can be used to overcome stress and for personal growth.

Goleman, Daniel. *The Varieties of Meditative Experience.* New York: E. P. Dutton, 1977.

A brief look at eleven systems of meditation and their practical applications.

Murdock, Maureen. *Spinning Inward: Using Guided Imagery with Children.* Boston: Shambhala, 1987.

Using guided imagery exercises with children.

Samuels, Mike and Nancy. *Seeing with the Mind's Eye.* New York: Random House, 1975.

A complete guide to the history, techniques, and uses of visualization.

Schwarz, Jack. *Voluntary Controls: Exercises for Creative Meditation and for Activating the Potential of the Chakras.* New York: E. P. Dutton, 1978.
Meditational exercises for controlling the body and its bioenergy.

Starker, Steven. *F-States: The Power of Fantasy in Human Creativity.* North San Bernardino, California : Borgo Press, 1985.
The productive role of daydreaming, imagery, and visualization in our lives.

Watkins, Mary M. *Waking Dreams.* Dallas, Texas: Spring Publications, 1984.
A Jungian look at the uses of mental imagery for self-understanding, with emphasis on the subject in historical perspective.

White, John (editor). *What Is Meditation?* Garden City, New York: Anchor/Doubleday, 1974.
An anthology of writings on different aspects of meditation.

VI. RELIGION AND SPIRITUALITY

Bach, Marcus. *Spiritual Breakthoughs for Our Time.* Garden City, New York: Doubleday, 1965.
A somewhat dated look at the rise of "experiential" religion and religious practices, but still informative.

Braden, Charles S. *Spirits in Rebellion: The Rise and Development of New Thought.* Dallas, Texas: Southern Methodist Press, 1987.
A complete history of the rise of New Thought philosophy.

Cohen, Daniel. *Close Encounters with God.* New York: Pocket Books, 1979.
A popular presentation of some of the research collected by Sir Alister Hardy and others on religious experience.

Gilmore, Don. *Extra Spiritual Power.* Waco, Texas: Word Publishers, 1972.

Developing extrasensory perception within a Christian framework and its relation to prayer.

James, William. *The Varieties of Religious Experience*. Reprint. New York: Random House (Vintage), 1990.
The classic on mankind's encounters with the numinous.

Kelsey, Morton T. *Psychology, Medicine and Christian Healing: A Revised and Expanded Edition of Healing and Christianity*. New York: Harper and Row, 1988.
A comprehensive, scholarly yet readable history of the role of healing in Christianity.

O'Brien, Elmer (editor). *Varieties of Mystic Experience*. New York: Mentor, 1965.
Writings of the great mystics presented in a popular format.

O'Brien, Justin. *Christianity and Yoga: A Meeting of Mystic Paths*. New York: Penguin Books, 1989.
A brief but scholarly look at the way Christian practices and yoga share certain commonalities.

Parker, William R. and Elaine St. Johns. *Prayer Can Change Your Life*. Englewood Cliffs, New Jersey: Prentice-Hall, 1983.
An experiment in self-healing through prayer carried out in Redlands, California .

Weatherhead, Leslie D. *Psychology, Religion and Healing*. New York: Abingdon Press, 1952.
A classic book on the interface between psychology and religion.

REFERENCES/CHAPTER NOTES

NOTES

INTRODUCTION—SPIRITUALITY, HEALTH, AND THE MIND

Achterberg, Jeanne. *Imagery in Healing: Shamanism and Modern Medicine.* Boston: Shambhala, 1985.

Achterberg, Jeanne, et. al. "Psychology of the Exceptional Cancer Patient: A Description of Patients Who Outlive Predicted Life Expectancies." *Psychotherapy: Theory, Research and Practice: 14,* 1977, 416–422.

Braden, Charles S. *Spirits in Rebellion: The Rise and Development of New Thought.* Dallas, Texas: Southern Methodist University Press, 1987.

Deleuze, J.P.F. *Practical Instruction in Animal Magnetism,* Reprint. New York: Da Capo Press, 1982.

Ellenberger, Henri F., *The Discovery of the Unconscious: The History and Evolution of Dynamic Psychiatry.* New York: Basic Books, 1981.

Frank, Jerome D. *Persuasion and Healing: A Comparative Study of Psychotherapy.* New York: Random House (Schocken), 1963.

Fuller, Robert C. *Alternative Medicine and American Religious Life.* New York: Oxford University Press, 1989.

Fuller, Robert C. *Mesmerism and the American Cure of Souls.* Philadelphia: University of Pennsylvania Press, 1982.

Klupfer, Bruno. "Psychological Variables in Human Cancer." *Journal of Projective Techniques: 21,* 1957, 331–340.

Peel, Robert. *Spiritual Healing in a Scientific Age.* San Francisco: Harper & Row, 1987.

Podmore, Frank. *From Mesmer to Christian Science.* Reprint: New Hyde Park, New York: University Books, 1963.

Rossi, Ernest L. *The Psychobiology of Mind-Body Healing: New Concepts of Therapeutic Hypnosis.* New York: W. W. Norton, 1986.

Silberger, Julius. *Mary Baker Eddy: An Interpretive Biography of the Founder of Christian Science.* Boston: Little, Brown and Company, 1980.

REFERENCES/CHAPTER NOTES

CHAPTER 5—EXPLORING THE CREATIVE MIND

Harman, Willis and Howard Rheingold. *Higher Creativity*. Los Angeles, California: Jeremy P. Tarcher, 1984.

Rogers, Carl. *On Becoming a Person*. Boston: Houghton Mifflin Co., 1972.

Terman, Lewis M., et. al. *Genetic Studies of Genius. Volume I: Mental and Physical Traits of a Thousand Gifted Children*. Stanford, California: Stanford University Press, 1925.

Terman, Lewis M. and Melita H. Oden. *Genetic Studies of Genius. Volume IV: The Gifted Child Grows Up*. Stanford, California: Stanford University Press, 1947.

Terman, Lewis M. and Melita H. Oden. *Genetic Studies of Genius. Volume V: The Gifted Group at Mid-Life*. Stanford, California: Stanford University Press, 1959.

Wallis, Graham. The Art of Thought. London, 1926.

CHAPTER 10—CAN PSYCHIC HEALING BE LEARNED?

Ebon, Martin. "Russia's Superhealer." *Fate, 35* (#8), 1982, 39–44.

Gris, Henry and William Dick. *The New Soviet Psychic Discoveries*. Englewood Cliffs, New Jersey: Prentice-Hall, 1978.

Hill, Scott. "Paranormal Healing in Russia." *Fate, 34* (#8), 1981, 60–69.

CHAPTER 14—MANKIND: PROGRAMMED FOR RELIGION?

Bear, David M. and Paul Fedio. "Quantitative Analysis of Interictal Behavior in Temporal Lobe Epilepsy." *Archives of Neurology; 34*, 1977, 454–467.

Beecher, Maury. "Three Cardiologists Report Prayers for Their Patients Are Answered." *Medical Tribune*, January 8, 1986, *1*.

Bucke, Richard M. *Cosmic Consciousness*. Reprint: New York: Carol Publishing, 1984.

Byrd, Randolph C. "Potential Therapeutic Effects of Intercessory Prayer in a Coronary Care Unit Population." *Southern Medical Journal: 81*, 1988, 628–829.

Collipp, Platon. "The Efficacy of Prayers: A Triple Blind Study." *Medical Times*, 97, 1969, 204.

Dewhurst, Kenneth and A. W. Beard. "Sudden Religious Conversions in Temporal Lobe Epilepsy." *British Journal of Psychiatry*: 117, 1970, 497–507.

Feldman, Robert G. *Neurology: The Physician's Guide*. New York: Thieme-Stratton, 1984.

Galton, Francis. *Inquiries into Human Faculty and Its Development*. New York: AMS Press, 1972.

Gardner, Rex. *Healing Miracles*. London: Darton, Longmen & Todd, 1986.

Gardner, Rex. "Miracles of Healing in Anglo-Celtic Northumbria as Recorded by the Venerable Bede and His Contemporaries: A Reappraisal in the Light of Twentieth Century Experience." *British Medical Journal*: 287, 1983, 1927–33.

Gazzaniga, Michael S. *The Social Brain: Discovering the Networks of the Mind*. New York: Basic Books, 1987.

Geschwind, Norman. "Interictal Behavioral Changes in Epilepsy." *Epilepsia*: 246 (Supplement 1), 1983, 523–530.

Hardy, Alister. "Research into the Spirit of Man." *Psychic*, September 1972, 24–27.

Hardy, Alister. *The Spiritual Nature of Man*. London: Clarendon Press, 1979.

Hay, David. *Exploring Inner Space: Is God Possible in the Twentieth Century?* London and Oxford: Mowbray, 1982.

Hickey, Des and Gus Smith. *Miracle*. London: Hodder & Stoughton, 1978.

James, William. *The Varieties of Religious Experience*. Reprint: New York: Random House (Vintage), 1990.

Joyce, C.R.B. and R.M.C. Welldon. "The Objective Efficacy of Prayer." *Journal of Chronic Disease*: 18, 1965, 367–77.

Loehr, Franklin. *The Power of Prayer on Plants*. New York: Doubleday, 1959.

Parker, William R. and Elaine St. Johns. *Prayer Can Change Your Life*. Engelwood Cliffs, New Jersey: Prentice-Hall, 1957.

Skutch, Robert. *Journey Without Distance*. Berkeley, California : Celestial Arts, 1984.

Waxman, Stephen G. and Norman Geschwind. "Hypergraphia in Temporal Lobe Epilepsy." *Neurology*: 24, 1974, 629–636.